Praise for *Shroomies*

"*Shroomies* is an important contribution to the research into psilocybin mushrooms and mental health. The book combines both a comprehensive study of mushrooms—dating back to when the earth was still forming—to the party era of hallucinogenic drugs—then finally revealing Biggs's own very personal and very honest journey in seeking help for his struggles with depression. He offers a strong testament and a path for others in understanding the powerful tool psilocybin mushrooms might have in their own recovery."

—Sharon Dilworth, author of *To Be Marquette*

"This is the book I didn't know I needed in my life."

—Dennis Walker, founder of Mycopreneur

"As someone with a bit of history with mushrooms of all kinds, Biggs has written an easy-to-read and heartfelt exploration of the magic kind. A fascinating read."

—Michael Azzolina Cecchi, restaurateur and author of *Your Table Is Ready: Tales of a New York City Maître D'*

"John Biggs writes like he's got nothing to hide—and that's what makes it hit. Part breakdown, part breakthrough, *Shroomies* is as honest as it gets."

—James "Murr" Murray, Impractical Joker and bestselling author of the *Awakened* trilogy

Shroomies

Shroomies

How Mushrooms Cracked My Heart Open—and What They Can Teach Us About Healing

JOHN BIGGS

Skyhorse Publishing

Skyhorse Publishing books may be purchased in bulk at special discounts for sales promotion, corporate gifts, fund-raising, or educational purposes. Special editions can also be created to specifications. For details, contact the Special Sales Department, Skyhorse Publishing, 307 Fifth Avenue, 4th Floor, New York, NY 10016 or info@skyhorsepublishing.com.

Skyhorse® and Skyhorse Publishing® are registered trademarks of Skyhorse Publishing, Inc.®, a Delaware corporation.

Visit our website at www.skyhorsepublishing.com.

10 9 8 7 6 5 4 3 2 1

Library of Congress Control Number: 2026940082

Cover design by Kai Texel
Cover image by Getty Images

Print ISBN: 978-1-5107-8381-2
Ebook ISBN: 978-1-5107-8382-9

Printed in the United States of America

Disclaimer

This book is not a guide to identifying or taking mushrooms.

Many psilocybin species have highly toxic and sometimes deadly lookalikes. Misidentification is common, even among experienced foragers in unfamiliar regions.

Do not consume any wild mushroom unless they have been confirmed by a qualified expert. Mistakes can lead to serious illness or death.

Consuming psychedelics like psilocybin without the assistance of a psychiatrist, doctor, or clinician is dangerous. Please consult with an expert before trying anything discussed in this book.

For Robert Biggs, who started this whole journey.

Contents

Author's Note

I've taken the liberty of using only the first names of many people in this book for various reasons. Mushrooms, in many places, are still illegal and it's important to protect the amazing people who work with, share, and experience these plants on a regular basis.

Most of what you will learn in this book will be illegal in your country or state. While all the information I offer here is publicly accessible online, please do not try anything you find here if you are in a place where growing or consuming mushrooms is prohibited.

I'm not a doctor.

If you are under psychiatric supervision or suffer from any mental health issues, please consult with your health-care provider before trying any psychedelic medicine. Please consume psychedelics safely, ideally in the company of a trained professional.

Chicago

It was 10:39 p.m. on a rainy May night in Chicago when I decided to walk in front of a city bus.

My father had died half a year earlier, in January 2018, after a short and violent fight with lung cancer.

"It was nice knowing you, son," he said, in a moment of clarity, before the hospice nurses gave him morphine. He slipped into organ failure, then unresponsiveness. Everything before that moment, the frantic trips from Brooklyn to Columbus, where my parents lived, the wheezing that worsened by the day, the hacking cough that brought up endless fluid, are seared in my memory. His last moments, the death rattle, still rise like dark bubbles and bring a knot to my throat.

He was a big, warm man, someone who could talk to anyone and who drank like a Greek god. I knew he was dying when he refused a glass of wine on Christmas Eve. He died the day after New Year's.

The cruel irony was that a man who loved to eat, a man who once weighed 425 pounds, was taken by a disease that made his lungs look like uncut Hormel deli meat and reduced him to an almost healthy weight. He labored and labored, taking experimental treatments and chemo at different hospitals. I would fly home to drive him to appointments, sitting with chipper doctors who said he had a chance.

Dad never had a chance.

He was stubborn. One night I yelled at him for drinking a beer, something the doctors had strictly forbidden while he was undergoing experimental therapy. The tables had turned. I was the one scolding my father, the man who had stood by me and, in his own way, shaped me through his mix of reprimands and praise. The father and son roles had reversed.

He grew weak, gaunt, distracted.

"Did you see the light outside today? The deer?" he asked me one afternoon in November. I asked him what he was talking about, and he shook his head as if clearing cobwebs.

"It was nothing, don't worry," he said.

But I was worried.

Fast-forward to the winter. He was coughing up sputum, dark and frightening. He couldn't breathe and he was on oxygen constantly. His face was thin and his eyes were small in his large head. I didn't recognize him.

I asked him to tell me stories from childhood and I recorded them. He rasped and wheezed, but he told me about his upbringing in Martins Ferry, Ohio, his mother who lost her first husband to black lung, his trips to Europe as a young bachelor.

He took to falling in the shower, and we'd have to call the fire department to lift him up. I couldn't manage him myself. I was too weak.

I remember his final moments, the silence after that labored breathing stopped.

I remember the grim comedy of dragging his still-massive body out of my parents' basement apartment, taking him up the elevator where we could barely move his weight. I remember speaking at the funeral, crying in front of friends and family who had come to carry him to rest.

I remembered it all, that whirling series of days where everything was wrong, everything came down on me like a blanket to smother my joy.

But of my night in Chicago, I can barely recall anything except a series of flashes. The pizza. The guitars. Drinks at a bar. The lights of the bus reflected in the rain. The drops breaking the scene into a thousand pinpricks. The dark street glazed with puddles.

That morning in May, I woke up feeling nothing. I was in Chicago for only two days. Over the years, as a constantly traveling journalist, I'd picked up a habit of flying into a city for the shortest time possible. It became a kind of challenge: How little time could I spend in a city, even after all the airport rigamarole?

Once, I landed in San Francisco, did a photo shoot with a B-list celebrity featuring some weird technology, and flew back home the same day. I told myself I did it to reduce the time I was away from my young family, but it was really an act of self-torture, an effort to suffer for my drinking, my late-night carousing, my efforts to outrun my body and mind. This trip was a bit longer, but not by much. I loved the feeling of travel, the strange ceremony of gate, lounge, seat, hotel, but I'd come to hate myself in all these strange cities.

After breakfast, I set out walking through leafy neighborhoods toward Lakeview, on my way to a company called Reverb, where I was supposed to interview the CEO. The buds were coming in, but it was still Chicago cold, rain gathering on the horizon. I was still a professional tech journalist then, and PR people were still my only close personal friends. They called me to invite me to parties where I drank too much and talked too loudly, and sometimes they even flew me to places like Switzerland and Seattle to see new products. It was quite a life. People wanted me to share my deep and abiding wisdom about business and start-ups. I was a charlatan at best, but they didn't know that and, thanks to a dose of ego, neither did I. All the places I worked, like TechCrunch, the *New York Times*, and Gizmodo, had made me something of a D-list online celebrity, but not as popular or as personable as figures like Grumpy Cat.

Reverb buys and sells used music gear, from guitars to keyboards to amps. These days, thanks to my bad habit of buying too many guitars, I love Reverb. But that day I felt put upon, forced to talk to someone more successful than me, someone who got to spend his days around guitars and music gear. I'd hit a sad, weird point in my career where I was jealous of start-up founders' successes even though I couldn't find business success of my own. If I was so smart, I kept saying to myself, why wasn't I rich?

The Reverb offices were a treasure trove of cool gear, stuff that had been commissioned through them to sell online. The CEO, David Kalt, was running the kind of start-up I wanted to build. It was a happy place to work, full of cool people playing with cool music gear. Again, I was jealous.

Talking to Kalt, I had the sense that I had failed, that everyone else had the right ideas, the right jobs, the right money. I had none of it, even after a decade and a half of being a tech journalist with bylines in most major outlets: *Wired*, *New York Magazine*, *Men's Health*. I was on a downswing, and I felt it, the lurch in my stomach as I approached the bottom.

The interview was uneventful. I recorded it, probably, but I do not have the recording anymore. We walked around the warehouse, looked at gear moving in and out, stared at some amazing instruments from every decade.

After the interview, I went for deep-dish pizza at a place called The Art of Pizza near the Chicago Music Exchange. After eating the entire fourteen-inch pie, I wandered down the street to Chicago's temple of Fenders and Gibsons, where my eyes glazed over, uninterested in anything. The normal me, the me from a decade before, would have been salivating over guitars that were beautiful and, thanks to my job at the time, in reach. But I felt nothing. I picked up a few, strummed them without interest, texted my friend Rob some photos.

"Nothing cool here," I remember saying to him. The irony was lost on me. Everything was cool, but I couldn't see it.

This version of me, the one wandering around Chicago on that rainy afternoon, was pushing three hundred pounds and traveling nearly two hundred days a year. I was writing about the start-up economy of a world trying to claw its way out of the 2008 financial crisis. By 2018, I was not even really a journalist anymore. I had left the best job I ever had with some of the best colleagues, to try to build start-ups on my own. My old outlet, TechCrunch, let me pretend to be a writer for a few years after I quit, giving me access to events where they would fly me out, put me in a hotel, and get me drunk until I hit the stage. Onstage I was surly and uncomfortable for about thirty minutes until I could get back to drinking.

Investors were throwing money at start-ups, and because of my ego, I thought I could grab some for myself. I wanted to become the hero of my own founder story. By 2018, I had failed twice. Once I raised and lost almost a million dollars. The other time I built an entire product that became wildly popular with a few thousand people but could not gain real traction. Now I was freelancing for the site I had basically helped build, and I was fast on my way to becoming irrelevant.

On that day in Chicago, I knew why I had failed so completely. I was incompetent, incapable, unworthy of success. I was a lumbering oaf, too distracted to get anything done except write five-hundred-word articles about guys who were making more money and getting more praise than me.

I was a real treat to be around.

That night in Chicago, I had been invited to run a pitch off between multiple start-ups. These were new companies just taking off and, thanks to the way the start-up market works, many of them would fail. In that theater of entrepreneurship I was in, you were not supposed to talk about that. You were supposed to be openly enthusiastic. I was not. The pitch off was unmemorable, more companies that would never climb out of the swamp of the Chicago start-up scene, but they had an open bar.

I found myself in a pointless argument with a guy who had apparently been CTO of Barack Obama's 2012 campaign. I was petulant, angry, and drunk, after finishing a huge beer at the pizza place and then polishing off glasses of free wine at the event. The debate, centered on which city was more entrepreneurial, was trivial. Fights like this were becoming more common for me. My face was blank. My tone was mean. I was not being a nice person.

The problem was inside me. I was broken and angry. New products all felt the same. The start-ups I talked to were churning out copy-paste businesses. Scooter companies. Car-sharing clones. Apps to find your friends in a crowded club. I was exhausted. I could fly to Chicago and see the same lineup I saw in Tokyo and then fly to San Diego and see another fifty of the same start-ups. I had been writing about tech since 2000, and by then I had seen enough.

Also, my first reader, the man I wrote for, my father, was dead. When I banged out a TechCrunch post or a *New York Times* article, I was writing for him. He had been an English teacher turned government worker turned Rush Limbaugh Republican, and he was the person I was speaking to when I wrote for the world. He was someone who needed to hear about the latest thing so that the despair innate in his politics would not drag him under. I wanted to show him that, despite everything he heard on AM radio, the world was getting better. But he was gone.

So, there I was, fatherless, alone in a damp, chilly city, angry at the world. I had overeaten that day and I was drunk. I felt as large as my father had been and I wanted to be as dead as he was. A bus approached Elm Street just as I left the historic Biggs Mansion, no relation, where I had smoked a cigar with some friends. They had picked that spot with me in mind, a Biggs in the Biggs.

At 10:35 p.m., I was trying to find my way back to my hotel, pecking at my phone for a map. Then my brain broke and something told me to look up.

By 10:39 p.m., I had decided that all it would take to end this day was to step into the path of the number 70, approaching the corner of Elm and Dearborn. The lights inside the bus were as bright as day, and I remember seeing the driver's face, his eyes a passive mask at the wheel.

By 10:40 p.m., I was ready to take that step. Then I looked again at the driver. He was caught in the harsh light of that massive machine, eyes half closed, just doing his shift.

I felt sorry for him. He did not need his night ruined.

That thought stopped me. The thought that this poor driver would end his night slamming on the brakes too late, the clunk, the screech. A driver haunted by the memory of the fat fool who threw himself into his night, ruining it forever.

I was not thinking about my family, my kids, my wife, my mother, or my sister. I wasn't thinking about my father.

I wasn't thinking about myself.

I was thinking about this unnamed bus driver.

By 10:41 p.m., I understood that while he might get a few days off if I went through with it, the moment had passed.

I called a psychiatrist the next day.

I am not unique. In the United States, about 14.2 in every 100,000 people died by suicide in 2022. The age-adjusted rate for males was 23 per 100,000, compared with 5.9 for females.[1] I was one of the sad dads, part of a crowd of men who felt their best years were behind them and ahead, except those years, the years between diaper changes and retirement, were tearing them apart. I spoke to a friend's wife whose father had killed himself when she was in her teens. She never forgave him.

"You realize that if you kill yourself, all of us will suffer. We'll all be investigated for murder, the police will come after us," warned another friend later when I told him about my evening in Chicago. "It's a selfish act."

Slowly, slowly I pulled out of the spiral.

Who was I to complain? I was where I wanted to be, where I was supposed to be. My career was stable. I was a minor internet celebrity. At my tech blog, which drew 100 million page views a month, people knew who I was. They sought me out, hoping for a mention that could lift them from the trenches to dreams of Uber or Facebook money. Yet I was not seen as a person, only as a chance.

That was the curse. I had thousands of acquaintances worldwide but no one I could rely on or confide in. I could announce my arrival in a city and draw a hundred people to a bar, where I would outdrink them while talking about start-ups. People pitched me in bars, hotels, even bathrooms, cornering me at urinals. They wanted my attention, and I still felt like a failure.

My suicide attempt was a wake-up call to myself. I knew I needed help. My psychiatrist, whom I nicknamed "the Thing" for his calm way of speaking and his size, said I needed medication. I did not argue. I did not know any better.

For most of two decades, I had been on autopilot. My head felt empty of drama or regret. I said whatever I wanted in a way that was probably deeply insulting, and no one called me on it. I filled rooms with gloom and anger. I thought I could get away with it because I was a journalist, a teller of truths. It was their fault if they did not want to hear it. I did not care if what I said hurt.

I did not see that I was the one being hurt. Everybody else was just happy to get an article and then forget about me. I was the obstacle between them and their next million-dollar investment.

I started taking desvenlafaxine, an antidepressant that the Thing said would be mild and pleasant. I went all-in, gained a lot of weight, and waited for things to get better. The Thing and I did not do any talk therapy. I was too smart for that, or so I told myself. We just chatted for half an hour while he made sure the drugs were taking hold.

The meds worked, in a way. I was not falling apart. I was not crying in the shower. But I was not laughing either. I was not really anything. I had been turned down to a middle setting where nothing hurt too much but nothing felt good either.

Then the new problem started. I could not stop.

Missing a dose accidentally or deliberately was like yanking a wire out of my skull. The zaps would start, small electric shocks in my head, especially when I moved my eyes. It felt like flicking a loose cable behind a TV. Something in my brain said I shouldn't have been on this medicine, so I stopped occasionally but jumped right back on. Not because I wanted to, but because withdrawal was worse.

This went on for about a year. A long, gray, shapeless year. I showed up for work. I made small talk. I went to bed early and scrolled without thinking. I got through things. But I was not living in any real sense. I was stalled. I knew it, even if I did not want to admit it.

This could not be it. This could not be my only option.

This was not how I wanted to live. I needed something different.

Then I met the shroomies.

Unwashed Grapes

I hated Burning Man. I had never been, but I still hated it. I hated yoga music, that deep-throated chanting over sitars or instrumental versions of easy listening hits. I hated patchouli and flowing robes and drum circles and radiant people with 0 percent body fat who stayed well rested and spiritually complete on vegan diets. I hated hippies and hipsters and gazelle-like couples who danced equally well to techno and the Grateful Dead. I hated raves. I hated music. I hated fun. I wanted to stay home, read books, watch movies, and sink quietly into my own private malaise.

I told myself I had earned it. I had burned out as a writer, failed as an entrepreneur, and spent years away from my growing family chasing the high you get from open bars and business dinners. Nights ended in empty hotel rooms, drunk and stoned, waking at three in the morning to the sugar rush of metabolized booze and the anxiety of being alive.

I hated drug culture, the woozy potheads with vacant smiles, the acidheads, the candy flippers. I hated the new language of self-help, safe spaces, quests for self-discovery, bright smiles beaming up from a guru's feet. I was a skeptic, a follower of logic and fact, not interested in finding the shape of the universe or seeing the face of God.

I didn't like that people called LSD and peyote and ayahuasca "medicine." To me, they were drugs, and I didn't have time for them anymore after having sampled just a few of them in college. I had other stuff to do. It was like that guy in "Escape (The Piña Colada Song)." I was not into yoga, and I thought I had half a brain.

And yet, there I was, walking up a set of stairs into a beautiful, sunlit loft covered in psychedelic art, full of people for whom "vibing" was a verb. I was on my way to my first mushroom session, a twee-sounding event that involved lying around while listening to music. I was honestly angry. I considered myself above all this chanting, incense, and raga music. I had been a Taoist in college, whatever that meant, but now I was an atheist with a chip on his shoulder. A broken guy whose father had just died. A man who refused to accept that he was hurt, still grieving, and had lost someone vital to his well-being.

I was a guy who had almost walked in front of a bus and was, in some odd way, proud that he had mustered the courage to even think that dark, strange thought, a thought that grated like barbed wire on his brain. My brain.

I took off my shoes outside the room and went in. I found a spot on the floor against a wall, far from everyone else. My plan was simple: take the drugs, do what they asked, then leave as soon as I could. I had brought some unwashed grapes to share; I was told this was a potluck psychedelic session, and I dumped them on a counter crowded with vegan food and chocolate.

The apartment was one big, tall room with large bay windows facing the street. There were instruments up front: a gong, a guitar, a box that looked like a cross between a xylophone and a drum. Speakers were mounted to the walls and hidden in nooks. Every surface was covered in psychedelia and crystals. Sculptures were daubed in fluorescent paint, alien shapes glowing in the low light. Others were found-art pieces, like a bathroom full of bouncing rubber alien dolls. Everyone was settling in, preparing themselves. I sat with my back against the wall, waiting.

Traffic was roaring outside. Someone drove by blasting mariachi music, and a bus let off a head of steam under the windows. The loft was in the heart of the city, so it was revving motorcycles, police sirens, people shouting woozily at each other. It was as far from a Zen retreat as possible. To me it was just a rich guy's apartment outfitted with fuzzy pillows and massive crystals dumped into a nonworking fireplace.

The email I had received the day before told me to make a list of intentions. I was supposed to bring something comfortable to lie on, a sleep mask, maybe a totem to focus my mind. I was supposed to write a list of things I wanted to ask the universe, an idea I found absurd. I was not going to ask the universe for anything. It had taken a lot from me. Two businesses I tried to start. A career I loved, replaced by an endless hustle. It had taken my patience, my joy, and my father.

What else did I need? I was drinking often. I had a house and a family. Guitars and a few expensive watches. I told myself I had good taste in music and books. Most days I felt calm, helped along by a steady whiskey habit. All the important things, or so I thought. All the trappings of a Brooklyn intellectual. I wrote tweets, argued about politics on Facebook, and cranked out short pieces that few people read about things few people cared about.

I listened to jazz on vinyl, for Christ's sake.

The worst part was how feckless I felt, how useless. The one job I loved was gone, and I was cobbling together a living with gig writing and the odd full-time role that I always left after a year. When I quit my job at TechCrunch, I lost my tribe and my coworkers, and I did not want a new one. Time with those people had marked my happiest moments, when I was in demand, when my thoughts mattered. On that mushroom night, in a loft in late 2019, I saw myself as a nobody. If you had asked the people around me, they might have said otherwise. But the mind is a harsh scold. It pushes your nose into the dirt, and it makes you tally losses, not wins. It makes you think cruel things about yourself and those who love you.

Everyone there was prepared. They had big fluffy blankets and sachets of scented herbs. They wore formfitting yoga clothes and carried vegan leather notebooks that they would use to write down all their onrushing insights. I was not ready for this. I had a dirty sleep mask from a Delta flight and a sleeping bag. I brought my sweaty yoga mat and flopped it out to claim my space. I wore the coolest clothes I owned, black drawstring pants and a white Uniqlo shirt with something ironic on it. I nursed a light hangover and did not want to be there. I came to go through a mushroom session, something I did not care to do but had been nudged into by a well-meaning friend.

This friend, a guy from Nebraska named Greg, had always been a pain. When I met him in San Francisco, he was a tight coil of nerves. A muscular little nerd into the hardest core self-help, CrossFit, genome-based diets, local honey for inflammation. He was the kind of guy who prescribed blueberries from a specific farm ten miles away to treat a cold. People at work avoided him. He was odd. I was amused.

"Buy me ice cream," he would say as we wandered the Tenderloin in San Francisco. His diet (at that moment) called for late-night sugar to trick his metabolism. I laughed and bought us whiskeys that he handed back because his web searches told him alcohol caused sadness. Little did I know.

I envied him. I envied his drive to experiment, his faith in ideas that seemed silly. He read all the studies, did all the research, and came away certain that kettlebells and pureed kale would help him live forever. Who was I to argue?

My own research said I was a fun guy. I was great between beers two and five, annoying at six to nine, and amazing again after beer ten and the first gin and tonic. I was about three hundred pounds and healthy enough to outdrink most of my friends. I loved being the life of the party, loved the warmth of the first sip, hated the long night that followed, the ringing head, the rapid heartbeat, the late-night texts hunting for the next bit of fun.

I quit that job and lost touch with Greg when I stopped going to San Francisco. I was mad at everyone, so I did not reach out. One afternoon in October 2019, I ran into him in Brooklyn. The jittery guy was gone. In his place stood someone calm, steady, smiling. He tried to get me to smile. I did not trust it. What had changed?

We went to a bar. He said he felt better. He pointed to my beer and said, "Stop that." I laughed. That cold ale was my lifeline. It tasted great.

Then he told me his story. He said he got a new lease on life. He had suffered from chronic insomnia for decades. All his flailing in San Francisco, the diets, the workouts, the supplements, was about fixing that. The stuff we mocked was all about sleep and how he couldn't get any.

He found psychedelics. Not for fun. Not like in college. Psychedelics as medicine. He wanted answers and found them in a baggie of crushed psilocybin. A few years earlier he flew to Amsterdam for a mushroom retreat. There were no formal programs in the United States then, so he had to travel. He wanted a serious process, not a hippie-dippie sound bath. He wanted science.

They gave him mushrooms. The organizers told him to sit quietly and listen to music. None of it was mandatory, so Greg took some mushrooms and went to sleep. He slept for most of twenty-four hours. The next day he took more mushrooms and slept again. In the middle of that, the mushrooms told him he needed medical help.

"They told me I was sick," he said. He meant it. His body was talking back. It told him he had severe sleep apnea. While he slept, his throat closed, choking him. He would wake up, snort air, and fall back asleep. Repeat. Greg was not overweight. He was born with a nasal cavity that failed him. The mushrooms explained, yes, explained, that he needed to fix his nose. A doctor confirmed it. Massive occlusion. CPAP. Surgery. Years later, after over nine surgeries, he was finally healthy. He slept well, and he smiled at me with a glow that made me think he was on some experimental molecule.

The mushrooms saved his life.

After that, he became a psychedelic advocate. Plant medicine, he called it. He wrote reports and pushed for legislation. I had no idea this had happened. I only knew he seemed cooler now. Still nerdy, still Midwestern, but cooler.

I wanted that. I was taking pills I hated that made me gain weight. I woke up angry, cursing the day. I was driving my family away while hunting for something I had lost years before. Was it comfort? Respect? Control? I wasn't sure. I hoped mushrooms could help.

So, I said yes to the session. I showed up. I rolled out my sleeping bag. I kept quiet. More folks strolled in from the outside as the air conditioners hummed and sage wafted over the crowd. Everyone had an air of beatific calm. They greeted each other like old friends, commenting on their tans. They kissed on the lips, like this might turn into an enlightened orgy if they got the fat, grumpy guy out in time.

I did not expect much. Maybe a small trip, some fun. Like many Gen Xers, I never saw psychedelics as tools. I tried them once or twice, felt odd, and stopped. I tried LSD in college. I ended up curled on a friend's lap, saying I felt five inches tall. I never tried ecstasy during the rave years, even though I wore big pants and danced to drum and bass. I still smoked pot when offered but never took mushrooms. They seemed risky or, more precisely, too much of an investment.

That is not quite true. I took mushrooms once in The Hague. A friend and I made tea of specially purchased magic mushrooms at a Burger King and wandered the suburbs. We ate the soggy shrooms right out of the cup because we weren't sure how much to take. We went to a club, started dancing, and suddenly felt time stop. The club, for some reason, kept playing "The Chicken Song" repeatedly, and we were enthralled. What was this sorcery? Everyone was excited for the music, and we were convinced we were at a fourteen-year-old's birthday party. We fled the club, and I ended up back in my hotel, hearing techno in the HVAC and thinking about the length and breadth of Madonna's career while watching Dutch TV. It was a silly trip, signifying nothing. I expected more of that.

As the event started, we listened to the trip sitter. He was a mellow guy with long hair and an acoustic guitar habit. He had a calm voice and greeted each person, even me, the grump, with a handshake or a hug. He handed out our medicine, a baggie of mushrooms and a small dose of MDMA, and began by telling a story about heaven and hell as people settled in.

"A powerful samurai came to a small monastery and asked for the difference between heaven and hell," he said. "The monk looked him over, saw the blood on his armor and the mud on his boots, and said, 'You are a brute. I have no time for fools like you.' The samurai, enraged, drew his sword. His face went red. He was ready to kill the monk. The monk said, 'That is hell.' The samurai froze. He understood. His anger, his pride, his violence, that was hell. He lowered his sword and bowed. The monk said, 'And that is heaven.'"

It was a good story. I later learned it was part of his usual script. At that moment, however, I was drawn in. That story, trite as it was, meant something to me. This simple tale of a samurai and a monk made me think hard about where I was in life. I felt like I was in hell but in fact I was in a place of privilege with a bunch of nice white folks who weren't out to hurt me but instead wanted to listen to music and take some mushrooms. I was safe, I had enough money for this experience, and I was going to be okay. My head was making my own hell.

We each took half of a four-gram bag of powdered mushrooms. The sitter said it was Golden Teacher, a strong strain known to be gentle on beginners. I poured my share into my mouth and lay back with the mask over my eyes.

An hour passed. We did breathing exercises meant to calm the nervous system. The facilitator said the vagus nerve runs from the brainstem through the chest to the gut. It helps regulate heart rate, digestion, and mood. When parasympathetic activity rises, the body shifts from fight or flight toward calm. Chanting can help. Long, low sounds, like single, drawn-out notes or steady humming, vibrate the throat and increase vagal activity and heart-rate variability. It is not mystical. It is physical. It signals safety to the body. Many religious traditions use chanting, the most familiar being the "om" in Buddhism.

We took two more grams and some MDMA.

About six hours later, I came out of a meditative state, the most joyful I had ever known.

In that meditation, I flew through a fractal tunnel that folded on itself like origami made of light. I saw castles of color and faces smiling at me through vines of neon green. I became sound, became breath, became a dot of light that grew to infinity and back. The music was alive. Notes and rhythm and timbre made new sense. It carried me through the hours like a silver boat on dark water. I still remember every note of Leon Bridges's "River," as if it were played inside my bones, each breath and each guitar slide bursting like fireworks in my mind.

The song hit hard. Something cracked. Like the Grinch. Like Scrooge. Like a cartoon figure curled tight with anger that suddenly stretched out. My chest opened. I breathed, finally.

I felt okay.

The MDMA capsule, explained the trip sitter, was a buffer for the intensity. It did not make things happy. It made them kinder. It made the mushrooms put on a warm sweater.

I cried. Quietly. Not sobbing. Just tears. They rolled without warning, like someone turned a valve. I saw my father. I heard his voice, not booming with anger, but soft, like when he explained things to me as a kid. He told me I did not have to be sad. That I did not have to carry all this anger and shame and guilt.

I believed him.

Later, we did a scream session. We opened our mouths, stretched, and howled. It was silly. It was primal. It felt foolish and freeing at once. Then we shouted love into the world. Again, silly, but I meant it. For a moment, I meant it.

We were told to visit our inner child. We had to picture a wide field. A tree. A small version of me under it. *Go to him. Hold him.*

I did.

Big, grumpy me walked up to that tiny kid in my mind, sitting alone with knees to chest, and picked him up like I pick up my own kids. I held him. I told him it was okay. That he was okay. That he could stop being afraid. That he could stop being sad. That his dad was dead but that it wasn't the end.

It sounds corny. I know. It's amazingly hard to talk about psychedelic trips narratively simply because they are above narrative. It sounds silly, ridiculous, like a dream after some bad cheese. Six hours earlier I would have mocked it. I did not mock it then. Something had shifted.

That night changed me.

The changes didn't come all at once. I did not wake with a new personality or a six-pack or a certificate in advanced love. But something opened. Something softened.

I started to feel again.

That is the part few explain about depression. It is not only sadness. It is numbness. A fade into apathy. A gray fog that mutes everything. I lived in that fog for years. The mushrooms pierced it.

After that night, I was curious. Not only about psychedelics, but about why they worked. Why did psilocybin make me feel okay for the first time in years? Why did it help when therapy and pills and booze did not?

I started reading. Then I started growing. My kids called the jars in the basement our smelly mushroom roommates, our shroomies. The basement smelled like loam. I leaned into the lore of mushrooms and learned how to grow them in the same way I used to make wine and beer. I became the neighborhood mushroom guy.

I took them on a schedule. Not to get high, but to stay even. Small doses. Enough to take the edge off without drifting into bright colors. I started therapy. I drank less. I slept better. I was calmer. I was kinder. Slowly, I came back.

And I still had questions.

Why do these odd fungi, with names like Penis Envy and Jedi Mind Fuck, work so well? Why do they help with grief, trauma, depression, and self-hate? Are they really medicine? Could they be better than the pills I took for years? Are they dangerous? Or was I taught wrong?

I am a journalist. When something confuses me, I ask questions.

That is what this book is about. How mushrooms are changing lives. How they changed mine. How they help our minds, ease grief, and remind us to be human. It is about people, scientists, therapists, growers, skeptics, trying to understand what these ancient organisms offer.

I chose to grow eight strains, from Golden Teacher to Jedi Mind Fuck. I tried Blue Meanies. I grew the infamous Penis Envy. I talked to people who heal with mushrooms and people who warn against them. I tried to learn what happened to me in that dumb loft.

For this book, I talked to almost a hundred people about their mushroom use. Most shared the same arc. They were down. They were in trouble. Mushrooms helped them back up. They reopened faith and love, helped rebuild ties, pulled people from deep depressions. They taught people to take pleasure again, helped with recovery after loss, and helped one woman sing and dance after years of early onset dementia. They helped people live, and they helped people die.

They helped me.

This is the story of how mushrooms cracked my heart open.

It is also the story of how they might do the same for you.

Meet the Shroomies

Before we get into growing, tripping, or healing, we must go back. Not to the 1960s or a mushroom retreat last year, but way back before humans, before forests, before anything with a spine. Because before we start eating mushrooms or asking them to fix our lives, we need to understand what they are and where they come from.

Shroomies aren't just unusual plants or psychedelic tools. They're not even plants. They don't photosynthesize or make their own food from sunlight. Instead, they consist of underground mycelium that releases enzymes that break things down in the soil, digesting whatever it can find and turning it into fuel.

Mycelium is the fungus itself, a living body hidden in soil, wood, and leaf litter. Most mushrooms, the parts we can't see, consist of a fine, white web of string called hypha that threads through whatever it grows in, quietly digesting dead matter and returning it to the biome. It does not just clean up. At plant roots, mycorrhizal—literally mushroom and root—mycelium trades minerals and water for sugars, knitting life together. When conditions line up, that buried network sends up mushrooms, a fruit that releases spores and starts the whole story again. Unlike plant life, fungi don't have separate life stages or organs. Everything they are is right in the open, made up of mycelium, from the stringy hyphae to the woody truffle. They react almost mechanically to various stimuli but their entire tool kit, the Swiss Army knife of reactions they manage, is astounding.

They're also part of a vast, hidden network that has been quietly running the world for over a billion years. The biggest living thing on Earth isn't a whale or a redwood. It's a mushroom. Or more accurately, it's a massive underground individual of a species called *Armillaria ostoyae*, also known as honey fungus, growing beneath the Malheur National Forest in eastern Oregon.

You wouldn't notice it at first. Aboveground, it just looks like a scattering of small yellow-brown mushrooms poking out of tree stumps. But underground, it's something else entirely, a sprawling network of mycelium stretching over 3.5 miles, all part of a single genetic individual. It's the same DNA and the same organism, quietly expanding through the soil.

So, before we treat them like medicine, food, or some kind of spiritual shortcut, we need to see the bigger picture. What are mushrooms, really? What were they doing before we showed up? And what are they still doing now, quietly holding life together?

Let's start there. Let's meet the mushrooms.

Mushrooms are everywhere and have been everywhere for millions of years. Right now, they're all around you. We ingest them when we eat fungi on our pizza. And while we sleep, we breathe in small amounts of the fifty megatons of spores that mushrooms release each year. You can even wear them if you believe the proponents of mushroom leather, who say it is superior to bovine leather.

There are an estimated 2.2 to 3.8 million species of fungi on Earth, according to a 2017 study published in *Microbiology Spectrum* by David L. Hawksworth and Robert Lücking.[1] Of those, only about 150,000 species have been formally described. Some fungi just sit around forests, breaking down old trees. Others help us make bread, beer, cheese, and medicine. And yes, some can kill a human in a matter of hours.

Fungi are the quiet, behind-the-scenes medics of living systems. They recycle dead material, unlock nutrients, and stitch soils together.

Fungi also act like a planetary immune system, breaking down what is spent, feeding on what is growing, and setting limits on what overruns the rest.

Underground, threadlike hyphae knit into mycelium that can span meters or more. Through mycorrhizal partnerships, this network links roots and helps move resources where they are needed. Experts call this the "wood-wide web."[2] Experiments show that carbon, nitrogen, and signaling compounds pass between plants through shared fungi in some settings and that trees use the network to signal other trees to danger and sickness. Researchers debate how widespread and purposeful this is across whole forests, but the effect is real enough in many systems to change which seedlings live, which trees recover, and how a stand responds to stress.

As I dove deeper into mycology, I always brushed up against the spirituality of mushrooms. Everyone said the same thing: Mushrooms created a network in the world and they did the same to our brains, connecting our synapses like taffy. As an atheist, I wanted to pull the shroomies subject away from world religions. I never met any gods or goddesses on my trips. I usually just met myself, in a form that was unrecognizable but immensely helpful. But as I watched mushrooms take root, expand, grow, reproduce, and then fall back into decay, I kept thinking about a strange book, *The Sacred Mushroom and the Cross* by John Allegro.[3]

We'll explore his unsurprisingly polarizing work later, but in essence, Allegro argued that early religious orders used mushrooms and mushroom symbolism, like virgin birth, rebirth out of death, and endless life, to create symbolic systems that might explain our own lives. That was interesting, but I dug a little deeper. Instead of seeing ancient Christians as a bunch of mushroom-worshippers, I saw mushrooms more like Shiva, the Hindu god who represents both creation and destruction simultaneously.

In Hindu tradition, Shiva isn't just the destroyer. He clears space for something new to grow. He breaks down what no longer serves. Mushrooms do that in nature. Fungi don't just live off death. They build from it. Same with Shiva. What looks like chaos or collapse is the start of renewal.

Both mushrooms and Shiva move between worlds. Shiva meditates at the edge of society, untouched by it, while also holding the power to shake it to its core. Mushrooms grow underground, hidden, but they change ecosystems invisibly and completely. Some can shift your mind. Some can feed you. Others can be turned into clothing or household items. Some can clean up hazardous materials. Either way, they're not flashy or showy or difficult. They just act.

And then there's the silence. Shiva doesn't speak much. Mushrooms don't either. They both wait, still and patient, until it's time to come to the surface in a glorious display of color, shape, and size. They communicate in strange and wonderful ways.

Back to the hard reality of soft mushrooms. Before my first experience, I had gone mushroom hunting only a few times, but I have often enjoyed the fruits of others' labor. My family comes from Poland, and the Poles are inveterate mushroom hunters. Every summer and fall, they head into the woods with baskets, knives, and an encyclopedic knowledge of edible species, gathering what always seemed to me an endless supply of delicious shroomies they'd fry up with butter.

The woods outside Warsaw are thick with porcini, chanterelles, and even a strange mushroom called *Mleczaj rydz*, the saffron milk cap, whose Latin name, *Lactarius deliciosus*, hints at its culinary delights. Fried in butter or pickled in brine, these mushrooms are a treasured part of Polish cuisine.

One autumn evening I visited a relative in Rypin, a small town in the Polish countryside. She had just come back from picking *borowiki*, large wild mushrooms that go by the scientific name *Boletus edulis* and the English name Penny Cap. These large, comical things looked like something an elf would hide under but when cut into risotto or stewed in soup they added that unmistakable frisson of conifer forests and woodsmoke. They were a distillation of the night, something delicious and unique to that small kitchen in a cold country.

But pick the wrong mushroom, and the results can be deadly or at least uncomfortable.

I distinctly remember one evening when my father came back to our suburban Ohio home with a mess of wild mushrooms he had found. He confidently fried them up and ate them. Within an hour, my dad, that big, tough guy who weighed in at three hundred at that point, was stricken by gut pains. We rushed him to the hospital, where they pumped his stomach to prevent worse damage. He recovered, but it was a reminder: Even experienced foragers can make mistakes.

Sometimes, the toxic compounds have nothing to do with humans at all. A mushroom's chemical defenses might have evolved to deter a fungus-eating beetle or another competing microorganism, but because our cells share some basic functions with those smaller organisms, the toxins end up harming us too.

The tricky part is that edibility or toxicity often comes down to very small differences. Two mushrooms that look nearly identical might have completely different chemical profiles. *Amanita phalloides*, the death cap, can grow in the same woods as edible *Agaricus* mushrooms. Sometimes they pop up only a few feet apart. One can feed you. The other can kill you.

Death cap poisoning also plays a nasty trick with time. You often feel fine at first. Symptoms can take six to twenty-four hours to show up. Then it turns into days of misery, and if treatment is too late, liver and kidney failure can follow.

In short: Mushrooms are edible when their biochemistry aligns with our biology, and poisonous when their defenses, designed for a very different purpose, happen to hit our bodies where it hurts.

Other mushrooms designed their life cycles to constantly thwart discovery. For example, during a trip I took to Croatia to hunt for truffles, a friend and I stopped at a place called Karlić in Buzet, just north of Lake Butoniga and south of the hilltop town of Paladini. The family there has been hunting truffles for generations. The countryside was covered with woods and there was a muck to the ground that meant the shroomies growing there would have plenty of liquid with which to expand.

Truffles are underground fungi that live in symbiosis with the roots of certain trees, especially oak and hazelnut. They develop as the fungus and tree exchange nutrients through a network of fine mycelial filaments in the soil. Rather than being planted like crops, truffles appear naturally after years of slow growth in the right soil and climate. That said, there are ways to help them along. The team at Karlić brought in pre-inoculated trees and root balls to cultivate truffles, but the old hunters still prefer the natural ones, the little surprises growing deep underground.

As we walked through the woods around Karlić, we were told we weren't seeing every inch of their land or trails. Truffle hunters, who can make hundreds of dollars from one pungent little mushroom, protect their favorite spots like gold prospectors or fishermen.

That afternoon, we took out one of their Lagotto Romagnolo dogs, Bubica, who was a little sister to two other curly-haired truffle dogs named Dalma and Bobza.

Lagotto Romagnolo dogs are curly-coated, medium-sized dogs from the Romagna region in Italy. Originally bred as water retrievers, they later found their true calling in truffle hunting. They're smart, focused, and less distracted than typical hunting dogs. They're not in it to flush out and bite down on rabbits or squirrels. That makes them perfect for the slow, deliberate work of sniffing out truffles. In places like Croatia, where the trade depends on precision, they've become the breed of choice, replacing the pigs that were often better truffle hunters but had a tendency to eat the goods if the handler was too far away to stop them.

Halfway through the tour, little Bubica, tail shaking and nose twitching, found a spot she liked. Luka, the truffle hunter, a dark-haired guy with a nose for mycelium, pulled out a knife and gently dug up a truffle about the size of a large jawbreaker. Priced at around $120 per pound, that little truffle would've earned about $80. Quite a haul for Bubica and, as I learned later from Rowan Jacobson's book *Truffle Hound*,[4] probably staged for my benefit.

But what fascinated me more was how Bubica found it and why truffles grow underground in the first place.

Truffles act like a second root system, a vascular counterpart that lets healthy trees feed weaker ones and allows the entire forest to sense drought, fire, or disease. To do that, truffles spend most of their lives underground.

The reality of these underground mycelial networks is far more interesting than any fanciful story about mushrooms letting us see God or gods because they are so interconnected.

Researchers have shown that in homogeneous tree populations, the mycelium of another truffle-like species (*Rhizopogon*species) physically links the root systems of Douglas firs (*Pseudotsuga menziesii*). In an amazing experiment, scientists introduced radioactive carbon-14 into one tree. Over time, they tracked how the sugars produced via photosynthesis in that tree moved underground through the mycelial network and entered neighboring trees' root systems.[5]

This experiment proved something critical: The network is not just a passive presence. It actively transports resources like carbon, water, and minerals between plants, helping to balance ecosystems and support weaker members of a forest community.

Because they fruit underground, truffles depend on animals to disperse their spores by crunching the hard truffle nodules or pooping them out. To lure them, they release potent volatile compounds that diffuse up through the soil. Specially trained dogs can detect these scents, earthy and musky notes shaped by species, age, soil, and microbes, and guide hunters to the spot with striking accuracy. Interestingly, according to Jacobson, humans can even snuffle out a truffle given enough effort. Particularly interesting was this exchange between Jacobson and a truffle hunter named Matteo. In this scene, the author goes traipsing through the woods with Matteo who is following a wet dog while brandishing a *vanghetto*, a small spade with small steel head and a long, tapered handle.

> That's our pattern. The dogs lope ahead, then dart to a random spot and start digging so often that we spend most of the next hour

in a full sprint, Matteo waving his arms at the dogs but daring not shout. Eventually I forget we're truffling at all. It's more like we're just out for a weird run with the dogs, kind of nice, actually. The rain has ceased, the blood on my cheek has dried, and I'm trotting through Tuscany with a crazy man. No complaints.

And so I don't even notice when Artu starts digging harder with his paws and doesn't chuff. But Matteo notices, and he barrels across the turf in his camo like a recruit in basic training. He yanks Artu away, falls to his knees, plants his face in the hole Artu has begun, and squeals. "Yes, here!" he says, lifting handfuls of dirt to his nose like a cokehead. "Smell! Smell!"

I kneel beside him and stick my own nose in the hole. It smells like dirt. "Are you sure?"

"Yes, yes!" He eases his *vanghetto* into the hole and scrapes away a millimeter of dirt. "Smell!"

I lean in. I smell dirt. Grass. Moldy leaves. And then, peeking out of the interstices . . . a tickle of garlic? "I don't know," I say.

"Yes, yes!" he says again, pushing me aside and resuming surgery. Artu tries to dart in and help, but I pull him back. Matteo leans in and squeals again.[6]

Unlike other mushrooms that push fruiting bodies aboveground, truffles have evolved to stay hidden. This strategy protects them from drying out or being eaten too soon. It also reinforces their relationship with the trees above. Like most fungus, they thrive through mycorrhizal symbiosis with specific trees including oak, hazel, and beech. That deep-root connection can only happen below the surface, where the truffle wraps itself around the tree's smallest roots.

So, these tiny masses of fungal cells speak to dogs and pigs in ways we can't comprehend. Like invisible, stinky beacons, truffles call out when they're ready. And all they ask in return is simple: Take me somewhere new.

Why linger on truffles? Because, like our magic shroomie friends, they have tuned a set of tactics, techniques, and slow organic growth that lets them thrive in their forests while outsourcing spore dispersal to animals. The animal eats the fruiting body, carries the spores, and deposits them far from the parent, complete with a bit of fertilizer. That is efficient evolution, less energy spent on building tall stems and caps, more on chemistry that gets the job done.

"Fungi are the grand recyclers of our planet, the mycomagicians disassembling large organic molecules into simpler forms, which in turn nourish other members of the ecological community," wrote mycologist Paul Stamets.[7] As we said before, they turn barren wastelands into brand-new worlds. They help plants, trees, insects, and animals grow. They've been doing it for so long that some of the first large organisms on land were fungal. They were here long before we crawled out of the muck onto dry land.

But why do mushrooms exist at all?

First, we need shroomies. Without fungi, the planet would be buried in the unprocessed detritus of life: dead trees, fallen leaves, lifeless animals, all piling up in a slow-motion avalanche of decay. Mushrooms, through their expansive underground networks, extract the last bit of usable energy from anything that once lived.

Fungi, as Stamets said, are chemical wizards. They secrete enzymes that take apart lignin and cellulose, the tough scaffolding of wood, and they can help break down hydrocarbons in oil spills. Some species bind heavy metals, others tolerate radiation, and a few even seem to harvest energy in high-radiation zones. Working with acids and time, they weather rock and help set the stage for soil to form. From there, they feed forests, steady water cycles, and even nudge atmospheric chemistry through the way they store and release carbon.

In other words, fungi do not just recycle life. They make life possible. They turn death into nutrients, keep organic matter moving, and make sure nothing, no fallen tree or forgotten scrap, remains stuck forever. If fungi had not evolved early in Earth's history, the planet would have choked on its own debris. With them, the cycle is endless. What was once leaf, bone, or bark becomes soil, and from that soil new life rises.

Biologists count fungi among the oldest forms of life on the planet. In 2019, researchers discovered fossilized fungi in the Canadian Arctic that are roughly one billion years old.[8] Identified through the presence of chitin in their cell walls, a defining characteristic of fungi, these ancient specimens predate the previously known oldest fungal fossils by more than 500 million years. This places fungi not only as companions to early plant life but potentially as some of the first pioneers of terrestrial ecosystems.

More recently, around 460 million years ago during the Devonian period, often called the Age of Fishes, towering fungal structures began cropping up across the landscape.[9] These were not the small, ephemeral caps we're familiar with today. Some, like *Prototaxites*, reached twenty to thirty feet tall and several feet wide, dominating early ecosystems.

At the time, vascular plants were only beginning to establish themselves. Most of the land was barren, with a few mosslike pioneer plants clinging to riverbanks and swampy deltas. There were no forests, no flowering plants, and few land-dwelling animals beyond early arthropods.

Into that emptiness, fungi moved. They had no leaves, no chlorophyll, and no need for sunlight. They broke down rock and converted it into usable nutrients. They created the first thin soils. They partnered with primitive plants and formed some of the earliest mycorrhizal relationships, exchanging minerals for sugars and anchoring life's expansion from water to land.

These partnerships were foundational. Without fungi acting as the silent middlemen, plants would not have survived the leap to dry land. Fungi bootstrapped the terrestrial ecosystem. They prepared the ground for the green explosion that came millions of years later.

Early fungi were so large because they had access to abundant nutrients and water. They were the only game in town, and they made the most of it. They encouraged the birth of new life while Earth's hot, turbulent surface slowly cooled and changed.

In this way, mushrooms were not just passengers in the story of life on land. They were drivers. Their presence during the Devonian marks one of the most important yet often overlooked transitions in Earth's history. They helped shift the planet from a blue, watery world to a green one. Their underground networks transported nutrients and forged connections between species. They laid the groundwork for life as we know it.

Ancestors of those giant fungi remained vital long after the Devonian. The earliest vascular plants had no true roots. Fungi helped them extract nutrients from rocky soils by forming primitive symbiotic relationships. The fungus helped the plant absorb water and minerals, especially phosphorus. In return, the plant supplied the fungus with sugars produced through photosynthesis.

Early mycorrhizal plants included species like *Cooksonia* and *Rhynia*, some of the first vascular land plants. They were small, leafless, and lacked complex root systems. This exchange made life on land possible. Plants needed nutrients locked deep in the ground. Fungi needed carbon. Together, they created a system that let both thrive.

Over time, this shaped the evolution of forests and ecosystems. Fungi were not just helpers. They were builders. They made it possible for plants to colonize barren landscapes and lay the first green layers of Earth's biosphere. These relationships still dominate today. Over 90 percent of land plants form mycorrhizal partnerships with fungi.[10] These connections help plants survive in poor soils and played a crucial role in the colonization of land during the wet Devonian.

Mushrooms also thrive after mass extinction events. During the Cretaceous-Paleogene extinction, which wiped out the dinosaurs 66 million years ago, fungi flourished.[11] With forests decimated and organic matter everywhere, fungal spores surged in the fossil record. Their ability to digest wood and thrive in chaos gave them an edge. They reshaped the planet. They consumed the dead and cleared the way for mammals.

"Fungi have persisted through Earth's five major extinction events, each of which eliminated between seventy-five and ninety-five percent of species on the planet. Some fungi even thrived during these calamitous episodes," wrote Merlin Sheldrake in *Entangled Life*, one of the books that brought mycology into the spotlight.[12] After the Cretaceous extinction, the one that ended the dinosaurs and leveled forests, fungi moved in. With the world littered in dead wood, their numbers surged. They found fuel everywhere and set to work, turning fallen trees back into soil.

Many fungi naturally form fibrous structures that can be molded into almost any shape. Because they evolved to survive in harsh conditions, their chemical makeup is remarkably resilient. Once harvested, mycelium can be dried, pressed, or treated to create a range of textures, from soft and pliable to rigid and durable. The results are materials that closely resemble animal leather, polystyrene, and synthetic fabrics.

Mushrooms can also produce materials that mimic leather and plastic. Researchers and start-ups have discovered that fungi can be used to produce sustainable alternatives to common materials like leather, foam, and packaging.[13] The key lies in the mycelium, a nearly limitless resource that is strong, flexible, and fast-growing.

Mycelium is valuable in manufacturing because of its unique physical, chemical, and ecological properties. At the core of its usefulness is its ability to grow into dense, interwoven networks that can be shaped and cured into strong, lightweight, and biodegradable products. Living mycelium is dried into a material that can be as hard as plastic or as pliable as leather. Although they are currently expensive, we may one day be walking around in mushroom shoes.

One company, PLP Labs, has demonstrated 3D-printed, mycelium-based, wood-like composites, suggesting fungi could one day replace conventional building materials. Imagine a fourth little pig with a house made of mushrooms, a house that is cheap, light, and surprisingly strong and smells like a bowl of barley soup.

Ecovative, a player in the mycelium materials space, has developed scalable methods for growing fungi into packaging, insulation, bricks, and leather alternatives. According to biologist and author Merlin Sheldrake, their materials are "lightweight, water resistant, and fire retardant. They are stronger than concrete when subjected to bending forces and resist compression better than wood framing."[14] Ecovative also produces meat alternatives made from mycelium, including vegan bacon, now sold in grocery stores like Whole Foods.

What sets mycelium apart is not just its performance but its sustainability. It can be grown on agricultural waste, requires minimal energy input, and biodegrades fully at the end of its life cycle. In essence, mycelium offers a living alternative to synthetic materials. Its chemical resilience, structural strength, and ecological compatibility make it one of the most promising materials for circular, bio-based manufacturing.

Fungal resilience extends far beyond product design. Fungi are vital to ecosystems and have demonstrated extraordinary abilities to survive in extreme conditions. One yeast species, *Rhodotorula taiwanensis*, thrives in uranium-contaminated environments and can endure intense acidity and radiation. Another, *Cladosporium sphaerospermum*, has been found growing inside the Chernobyl reactor, apparently using melanin to absorb and possibly metabolize radioactive energy.

In fact, scientists tested *Cladosporium sphaerospermum* aboard the International Space Station. A 21-millimeter-thick layer of the fungus was able to reduce radiation levels by approximately 2 percent, suggesting it could one day help shield astronauts on missions to Mars.[15]

Meanwhile, *Rhodotorula taiwanensis* continues to impress in high-radiation zones. It survives in acidic, metal-rich environments, forming biofilms in places contaminated with mercury, chromium, and aluminum. Some strains even consume cadaverine, the foul-smelling compound released by decaying bodies. These fungi are currently being studied for their potential in remediating toxic and radioactive waste.

Inside the human body, fungi are more than just guests. Some, like *Candida albicans*, are part of the normal human microbiome. They usually remain harmless but can shift into harmful forms depending on changes in the host environment.

Humans and fungi share molecular pathways and metabolic sensitivities, which may help explain why compounds like psilocybin interact so effectively with serotonin receptors in the brain. In some cultures, internal fungi are seen not as infections but as symbionts or entities that speak through the body and guide transformation. Whether seen as invaders or allies, fungi are already part of us.

To be clear, there are no mushrooms that can take over human brains and turn us into zombies. That remains fiction, at least for now. But fungi do control the minds of other creatures. The most famous example is *Ophiocordyceps unilateralis*, a parasitic fungus that infects ants.

It begins when a spore lands on an ant's exoskeleton and drills inward, using enzymes to breach its defenses. Inside, the fungus grows, spreading mycelial threads through the ant's body. Eventually, the fungus hijacks the ant's behavior. The ant leaves its colony, climbs a plant, and grips a leaf or twig at a specific height in what scientists call a "death grip." The host dies.

Then the fungus blooms. A fruiting body erupts from the ant's head, releasing spores onto the forest floor below, where new ants pass through. The cycle repeats.

Fungi like *Ophiocordyceps* do not just consume their hosts. They manipulate them. Research suggests they do not fully invade the brain but alter behavior through chemical signals that override neural control.[16] In some cases, such as infected cicadas, fungi even replace reproductive organs with fungal tissue. The insect lives on, spreading spores disguised as mating signals. It becomes a walking, flying fungal broadcast system.

These examples of parasitic fungi show how deeply fungi can entangle themselves with other species. They use the living, reshaping behavior and biology to suit their own ends. It is an unsettling mirror of the way shroomies can alter human consciousness with just a few grams.

Mushrooms have already shaped our ecosystems. To understand them is to understand the invisible scaffolding of life itself. They have been here longer than we have, they will outlast us, and in many ways, they've already taken over.

Why do they get us high?

The Wise Woman and the Banker

Now that we've met some of our shroomies' relatives, let's turn to the fungi we really care about: the magic kind, also known as *Psilocybe* mushrooms.

A mushroom is a mushroom, for the most part. *Psilocybe* mushrooms share this same fungal architecture as nearly every other mushroom on the planet but with one unusual trait. What sets them apart is a set of genes that build psilocybin from the amino acid tryptophan. Psilocybin is a secondary metabolite, so the fungus can grow and reproduce without it, but evolution has kept this pathway in several lineages, and in some cases even spread it by horizontal gene transfer, which suggests it offers some evolutionary advantage.[1]

Mushrooms produce a wide range of enzymes, acids, and small molecules that help them feed, defend themselves, and reproduce. Many wood-rotting species secrete powerful oxidative enzymes and organic acids into their surroundings to break down tough plant materials. Some mushrooms invest heavily in chemical defense. They make bitter or toxic compounds, including long-chain unsaturated acids, that reduce feeding by insect larvae and other small animals, and they also use toxins to compete with bacteria and rival fungi in the same habitat.

Psilocybe mushrooms follow the same general pattern. They live on organic matter and rely on the usual enzymatic tools to digest it, but they also carry a biosynthetic gene cluster that converts the amino acid tryptophan into psilocybin. The hard part is that we still do not have a single, clear answer for what that benefit is.

What we can say with confidence is that psilocybin is not made accidentally. It is costly to produce, and evolution has preserved and spread the genes for it, which tells us it has helped these fungi persist in the ecological niches where they live.

Could *Psilocybe* mushrooms be popular because they got our ancestors high? First, we have no real proof that animals experience psychedelic mushrooms the way humans do, only observations that some species consume psychoactive fungi and show behavioral changes, much in the same way, legend has it, that elephants can get drunk on the green fruit of the marula tree. So evolutionarily, there wasn't much need to produce psilocybin for most of mammalian history.

In fact, the only animals we can definitively say get high from a handful of shroomies are *Homo sapiens*.

Psilocybe mushrooms are globally plentiful. They grow nearly everywhere, including the pastures of England and Northern Europe, the veldts of Africa, and the grasslands of South America. They like earthquakes and mudslides and often thrive in disturbed places because disturbance exposes fresh organic material and changes light and moisture. Humans create lots of those conditions, from lawns to wood-chip mulch, so many species commonly fruit where we live. Shroomies spread via spores carried by wind, water, animals, and our landscaping, and we unwittingly introduce new species into strange ecosystems simply by opening a bag of mulch. In fact, we're probably the biggest reasons magic mushrooms grow anywhere at all.

"Psilocybe mushrooms and civilization continue to coevolve," Stamets wrote. "Today, many psilocybes are concentrated wherever people congregate, around parks, housing developments, schools, churches, golf courses, industrial complexes, nurseries, gardens, city parks, freeway rest areas, and government buildings, including county and state courthouses and jails!"[2]

From an evolutionary standpoint, then, we're looking at a fungus that grows simply because we like it. As we'll explore later, the reigning academic research suggests that shroomies grow because we want them to grow. In many cases, wrote Stamets, "guerilla" inoculations began appearing across the United States and Grateful Dead concerts became sources of raw mycelium for future grows.

"Private patches proliferated, as well as 'mushrooms-for-the-people' beds in public parks, arboretums, nurseries, zoos . . . virtually anyplace where sawdust was used. Public domain beds—planted or natural—attracted new enlistees and they, in turn, created satellite colonies. The result is a continually unfolding, exponential wave of mycelial mass. The yearly splitting and expanding of mushroom beds has created mycelial footprints from Washington to New York, from Arizona to Canada," he wrote.[3]

Currently, shroomies are one of the most widely available Schedule I controlled substances in the world, often found in urban environments and, as I learned, surprisingly easy to cultivate in a dark closet or basement. Anywhere humans go, shroomies are sure to follow.

I've only found magic mushrooms in the wild once. It was in the Hudson Valley in New York, the day after a cold rain. Mushrooms usually like warm rain, but these little guys were different. I parked along a stone wall where the road dipped past old orchards and horse pastures. The maples were turning the color of warm tea. Every surface held a thin gloss from the night's weather. I had come to walk, not to look for anything, but wet autumn grass has a way of showing you what it is hiding.

The field was a small town preserve with a loop path tramped by dog walkers and cross-country bikers. I cut off the trail where the ground sloped, and the soil went springy underfoot. The air smelled like leaves with a trace of wood smoke. In the low spots, the grass beaded with water. That was where I saw the shroomies.

At boot-sole height, scattered like thumbtacks, little bells rose out of the leaves. They were the color of straw dipped in tea, each with a pin-thin stem and a cap no bigger than a shirt button. They looked shy. I crouched down to look at them more closely. When I brushed a cap aside, the mushroom shed water in a clean, glassy sheet. They were most likely *Psilocybe semilanceata*, a.k.a. Liberty Caps, smallish mushrooms whose cute little tops made me think of Smurfs and clever wizards. I say most likely because I was no expert and identifying them was a skill that I didn't have. These Liberty Caps could have been something else entirely and consuming them could have killed me. That, obviously, is why it was quite a bit safer to grow these things at home.

I picked one but decided to leave the rest be. They were fresh, new, and probably needed to spread more than I needed to get slightly high. It was a joy, however, to see these odd little characters popping out of the detritus of the waning summer.

I was lucky to catch those Liberty Caps when I did, especially by accident. Real foragers know exactly when to go out. One friend told a story of a mycologist who checked the sky and weather at dusk and said, "We're going out tomorrow." Magic mushrooms often appear suddenly after a stretch of rain. They are mostly water, and what we see aboveground is the mushroom's fruiting body, an outgrowth of the hidden mycelium that is chock full of liquid. The mycologist could tell that a light rain overnight and then a warm morning would bring them out in droves. She was correct. They wandered the woods together and they found all types, including blue-bruising *Psilocybe* mushrooms of various species.

The mushroom lifespan is brief, a few days or less. The cycle starts as white, threadlike mycelium, the dense network that spreads through soil, wood chips, or mulch like ghostly roots. As the mycelium colonizes its substrate, it digests nutrients and prepares to fruit. Then, from the mat, tiny pinheads form, the first sign of developing mushrooms.

Each spike has the potential to become a "pin" or a tiny mushroom embryo. These pins emerge like little pegs from the ground, their heads still tucked tight, brown and rounded like matchstick bulbs.

Within hours, they begin to grow. What was a clean spot of mycelium at night can erupt by morning into a field of fully formed mushrooms.

When they reach maturity, they're a sight to behold. A box of homegrown mushrooms can feel like a magic trick. You spray the pins at night, turn out the lights, and wake up to a tub transformed, caps overlapping like shingles, their curved surfaces glowing in the UV light. It's a brief window of glory. The mushrooms bloom, their stalks stretch and firm up, and then, without warning, they begin to collapse. They drop their spores and melt back into the earth, softening, darkening, turning slimy in a matter of hours.

Mushrooms are also fickle. They won't grow in certain seasons, and you can spend hundreds of dollars on the best substrates, dirt, and systems and still not got a single mushroom. Unlike, say, a pepper seed, simply trying to grow mushrooms doesn't always get you a single mushroom.

But when they do grow, they explode.

More than once I've had to postpone a trip or rope a friend into babysitting just because I knew I'd miss the harvest window. Wait too long and you miss the chance to harvest. Personally, I was never able to pick my shroomies before they dropped their veils and spores, a no-no that many growers claim reduces the mushroom potency.

As for wild mushrooms, many of the best-known mushroom hunting spots were man-made, inoculated on purpose or by accident by a rogue mycologist in the wild. Many wild mushroom outbreaks are tied to a particular tree or even a particular gardener's buying habits. For example, Jochem Gartz wrote in 1972 that students at the University of Washington discovered the mother lode of mushrooms:

> During the fall of 1972, large numbers of a strongly bluing gilled mushroom with a distinct ring pattern were found at the University of Washington in Seattle. The fruiting bodies were found growing on bark mulch, which came from a central distribution point and which had been spread widely across the campus by gardeners. Due to the bluing reaction, students at the

> university assumed that the mushroom contained psilocybin, a belief that was confirmed later on. The sudden appearance of massive numbers of fruiting bodies quickly inspired students at the university to use the mushrooms as a hallucinogen.[4]

Once the students discovered mushrooms growing in the open, wrote Gartz, they doubled down on hunting for different species, encouraging the hunt along the rest of the Puget Sound.

"Redmond, WA used to be known as the bicycle capital," wrote Gartz. "Since 1978, several newspapers have renamed this city the psilocybin capital."[5]

In this case, the mulch could have come from the same forest of young trees and carried spores and mycelium from the chipper to the grass. Another researcher told me that an unnamed college spread wood chips imported from Australia on their grounds. The chips apparently had been inoculated with the wild by *Psilocybe* spores and the gardeners activated the mushrooms by spreading the mulch in the sun and watering the plants around them. Soon after the mycelium spread and matured, students found an endless supply of psychedelics that continued to pop up yearly as a kind of autumn surprise.

Mushrooms weren't always this popular. Until recently, these kinds of stories were rare. This is not because mushrooms were absent in the wild—they grew as abundantly as they do today—but until the 1960s a patch of fungus in the garden was seen as a nuisance or an interloper. Not many folks wanted to pick and eat weird shrooms and in a time before the internet and, more importantly, photography, it was hard to tell what you were potentially eating. That attitude held well into the 1950s. Some modern mushroom fans like to say people foraged them since the beginning of time to spark spiritual awakenings. The historical record does not support that, and in fact there are only a few clear mentions of psychedelic mushroom consumption in recorded history. While it is fun to picture early humans finding a patch of Liberty Caps or Golden Teacher and reaching transcendence, this probably rarely happened. Early humans would be meticulously careful about mushroom consumption. Picking and eating a weird shroomie was tantamount to suicide, especially given the fast-acting poisonous species they would have found in the wild. In practice, most people treated psilocybin species as dangerous, and serious efforts to classify, control, and study them only made them more popular.

Why all the horror stories? Start with risk. Eating any wild mushroom is dangerous. Many species look alike. Fly agaric, the red mushroom we will discuss shortly, shares a genus with killers like the death cap, *Amanita phalloides*, and the destroying angel, *Amanita virosa*. A single mistake could have been fatal for a forager on the savanna.

Timing confuses things further. Most plants that make people feel high act fast. Smoked cannabis can change mood in minutes. Alcohol has a slow and steady effect that anyone can track. Mushrooms often take an hour or more to come on and attack in a rush, resulting in a feeling of, at the very least, dread. Getting high on shrooms didn't help us take down mastodons. The other issue is that mushroom intoxication can give you an upset tummy. It's a real toss-up for a novice who might decide they were poisoned or cursed by a spirit of the woods. None of this erases the deep, careful traditions in which fungi were honored and used. It just makes clear those traditions were specific, not universal.

The notion that hunter-gatherers or ancient villagers would gladly ingest something that could incapacitate them for hours fails a basic test of survival. As Andy Letcher argues in his book *Shroom*, for centuries mushroom use was neither natural nor obvious. Popular stories about ancient peoples eating mushrooms to divine the future do not hold up to scrutiny.

"Of course, this kind of argument should immediately alert the critical enquirer," he writes. "Whenever anything is deemed 'natural' and 'obvious' it almost always turns out, on closer inspection, to be culturally specific, localized, and historically contingent. In other words, not at all natural or obvious."[6]

With the right set and setting—a wide-open beach house with comfy yoga mats and fluffy pillows—a mushroom trip can feel like a dream. In the dark woods of Paleolithic Earth, in a darkened Roman temple, or in the squalor of Victorian London, the same experience could feel indistinguishable from dying. It is hard to fend off bears when you are seeing mandalas of light while your fingers, as one person described on an ill-fated trip, seem to turn into snakes.

In that sense, today's magic mushroom culture is modern. It draws on older threads, including Aztec healing traditions, Siberian tales of ecstatic warriors, and the grim narratives spread by those who tried to suppress mushroom use, from Christian zealots in Greece to Catholic friars after Cortés arrived in the New World. But our love of psychedelics is very new, primarily because we had already mined the depths of ancient spirituality.

Researchers, writers, and historians, often with a pro-psychedelic agenda, have assigned mushroom lore to images that might simply resemble mushrooms. One well-known Neolithic carving from Tassili in Algeria appears to show a mushroom wizard in a bee mask, his body studded with liberty caps. For decades, this image, in a modified rendering by psychedelic writer Terence McKenna's then-wife, Kathleen "Kat" Harrison, has been taken as clear evidence of a mushroom shaman, with whirling psychedelic feathers on his head and mushrooms sprouting from every part of his body. The original artwork is far less definitive, and many researchers now argue that the supposed mushrooms are arrows, oars, or flowers.

While it's hard to point to prehistoric mushroom use, we do have proof that ancient Aztecs used mushrooms in their rituals. One of the earliest actual mentions of mushroom use appears in *Historia de las Indias de la Nueva España*, written by friar Diego Durán in around 1581. Drawing from an indigenous source now lost to time, Durán told of the coronation of Aztec king Tizoc around 1481, describing it in terms that wouldn't sound out of place at a modern rave:

> And all the lords and grandees of the provinces rose and, to solemnize further the festivities, they all ate of some woodland

> mushrooms, which they say make you lose your senses, and thus they sallied forth all primed for the dance.[7]

The mushrooms, called Teonanácatl, or "Flesh of the Gods," were reportedly bitter and often eaten with sweet add-ons. Spanish colonist Toribio de Benavente wrote:

> During the feast, they consumed some black Teonanácatl mushrooms, which had the power to intoxicate, cause hallucinations, and even arouse lust. . . . They ate the Teonanácatl mushrooms with honey, and under their influence, they felt themselves enflamed. Some began to dance. Others sang, while others wept because they were drunk. Some were speechless, sitting as if absorbed in the gathering place. Others believed they were dying in their hallucinations; others saw themselves being devoured by a beast; others imagined they had captured an enemy in battle; this one would be rich; that one would have many slaves. After the intoxication, they talked among themselves about their hallucinations.[8]

Again, not all that different from Coachella.

Mesoamericans even had what are now called "mushroom stones," carved stone artifacts that likely served a ceremonial or religious role in these cultures, especially among the Maya and possibly the earlier Olmec. While they are not universally agreed upon in terms of function, many scholars believe they are direct evidence of ritual mushroom use.

These stones are shaped like mushrooms with a rounded cap atop a whimsical stem, and have been found in Guatemala, El Salvador, and southern Mexico. Some stems are carvings of deities, jaguars, toads, or even decapitated figures, suggesting symbolic or mythological significance. Their craftsmanship and ceremonial burial imply they held importance to their owners.

Though the Aztecs themselves did not leave behind direct references to the stones, the continuity of mushroom use in Mesoamerican religious contexts, especially among the Mazatec, Mixtec, and Zapotec, suggests a deeper, older tradition.

Critics have pointed out the lack of definitive archaeological context for many of the stones and caution against projecting modern psychedelic frameworks onto pre-Columbian artifacts. Still, many scholars agree that the iconography and contexts of the mushroom stones, especially their association with death, transformation, and divine communication, support the idea that psychoactive mushrooms were ritualized in ancient Mesoamerican religion.

In short, mushroom stones and ancient stories likely represent one of the earliest artistic or symbolic recognitions of shroomies and their role in ritual life. This is not to say we know much about how they were used in everyday culture beyond the writings of a few grumpy missionaries.

As we dig deeper, we also learn where mushrooms got the bad rap they maintained for centuries. After Cortés and the European invasion of Mesoamerica, shocked Catholic friars wrote endlessly about the violence and horror associated with mushroom cults and, sadly, theirs are the only firsthand accounts we have of many Aztec traditions.

For example, Duran also wrote about a celebration day dedicated to the mushroom in the month of Ochpaniztli, or "Sweeping," that happened between August and September. This feast day was associated with fertility. The celebration was quite brutal, and it ended, at least according to Duran, with a horrific mushroom trip:

> The Sacrifice ends, and the temple's steps remain bathed in human blood, all go to eat raw mushrooms, a food that makes everyone lose reason and leaves them in a state worse than if they had drunk too much wine; they were so drunk and devoid of reason that some committed suicide, and thanks to the power of these mushrooms, they presented visions, and their future was revealed to them, their demon spoke to them, while they were in a state of intoxication.[9]

Tales of bad trips continued to percolate through many cultures. *Psilocybe* mushrooms were frequently cataloged alongside poisonous mushrooms in foraging and naturalist guides, and it wasn't until the 1900s that they began to be considered edible.[10]

This meant that for centuries mushroom intoxication was typically met with alarm. Doctors in Victorian England often wrote of patients who ate mushrooms gathered from public parks, presumably fried or boiled, only to fall under a strange spell that passed after a few hours. The key point is the episodes were frequently classified as a poisoning, not a psychedelic experience. In one case recorded in August 1830 by Dr. D. O. Edwards, a down-on-their-luck family named the Bickertons arrived at Westminster Hospital after eating fried mushrooms they had foraged in Hyde Park and Kensington Gardens. According to Andy Letcher in *Shroom*, laborers often collected mushrooms from these areas to sell for "catsup," a condiment made from salted mushrooms, nutmeg, and other spices that resembled a brown paste.[11] Finding no buyers for what were certainly psychedelic Liberty Caps, the Bickertons ate their own stock.

After about an hour, the family experienced what Edwards described as "the highest hilarity" and a kind of "inebriation [that] proceeded from no ordinary cause." He treated them by inducing vomiting and applying a few leeches to their heads. By the next day, everyone, including four-year-old George Bickerton, had returned to their normal, downtrodden state.

In other words, stumbling upon a batch of psychoactive mushrooms wasn't seen as lucky, it was cause for concern. That all changed about a century later.

The modern psychedelic renaissance can be traced back to a reserved, square-jawed banker named Robert Gordon Wasson in the mountains of Oaxaca, specifically the town of Huautla de Jiménez in the Mazatec region. Born in 1898 in Great Falls, Montana, Wasson studied at the London School of Economics. After serving in World War I, he returned to the United States and worked as a financial journalist for the *Herald Tribune* before crossing into banking. He joined the Guaranty Company of New York, then moved to J.P. Morgan & Co., where he rose to vice president, a post he held until his retirement in 1963, long after he had become known, improbably, as the world's most famous banker/(untrained) mycologist.

In 1926, Wasson married Valentina Pavlovna Guercken, a Russian émigré training to be a pediatrician. She had grown up in a culture that revered wild mushrooms, gathering them each autumn with her family. Wasson, raised in a mycophobic America, was wary of fungi. This difference between them sparked what he would later call an "ethnomycological" investigation into how cultures embrace or reject mushrooms.

The origin story, often misremembered, did not begin in Mexico but on their honeymoon in the Catskills. While hiking through the woods, Valentina spotted wild mushrooms, dropped to her knees, and gathered them with delight, bundling them into her skirt. Wasson stood back, appalled, convinced they were poisonous. That afternoon marked the first step on a path that, decades later, would lead the couple to Mazatec *veladas*, or healing ceremonies, in Oaxaca and, indirectly, to the first wave of Western psychedelic exploration. Mazatec *veladas* are nightlong rites held in private homes in the highlands of Oaxaca, led by a *curandera* or *curandero*—a healer—and structured around prayer, chanting, and ritual. Sacred mushrooms, called *santos niños*, are consumed not for recreation but for diagnosis and spiritual repair, with the healer acting as an interpreter rather than a guide to visions. These ceremonies long predate Wasson's interest and were embedded in everyday Mazatec religious life, aimed at restoring balance between the individual and the spirit world.[12]

Back to the Catskills. Valentina's decision to pick and eat a mess of mushrooms from the forest was appalling to Wasson. After all, mushrooms were poison, all of them death caps in disguise. He refused to touch the meal she cooked and went to bed convinced she'd end up dead. But morning came, she was fine, and he was left wondering how two people could look at the same mushroom and see such different things. That question, namely why some cultures fear mushrooms while others revere them, became the seed of a lifelong obsession. The way the tale expanded over the years says a lot about Wasson himself. He had a reporter's instinct and a showman's flair: Facts were useful, but a good story was sacred.

Valentina brought with her an interesting set of beliefs that presumably originated in the Kamchatka region of Siberia. Among the indigenous peoples of Siberia, especially groups like the Koryak, Chukchi, and Chuvanians, *Amanita muscaria* or fly agaric was reportedly used ceremonially by shamans. The mushroom was a sacred intoxicant that could induce visions, allow contact with spirits, and heal. Consuming fly agaric let the shaman venture to other realms.

Fly agaric, often described as looking like a Smurf house, is the red-and-white-capped shroomie that grows nearly everywhere. It has long been a cultural curiosity, showing up in eighteenth-century travelogues that describe the strange rituals surrounding it. Many of those stories haven't withstood modern historical scrutiny, but even in Wasson's time they were compelling and, given how easily the mushrooms could be found after heavy rains, easy to test.

Incidentally, if you'd like to see a real-life example of a bear eating and definitely enjoying a bunch of *Amanita muscaria*, Jean-Jacques Annaud's 1988 film *The Bear* features a big, fuzzy cub chowing down on an amazingly large and lurid patch of the muscaria, which leads to the bear tripping out to the sound of 1980s synthesizer music. This, unfortunately, isn't the wildest thing we know about fly agaric.

First, many indigenous groups believed a broth made from the mushroom, steeped in milk, would lure and kill flies, a helpful feature in the murky steppes, where water pooled and livestock stank. In Russia, fly agaric is still called *mukhomor* (*мухомор*), literally "fly killer."

The most notable connection of ancient Siberians to their shroomie friends comes to us from the people of Chukotka. Figures called the *Liudi Mukhomory* or Amanita People feature prominently in their first millennium CE Pegtymel petroglyphs including a series of images featuring humans next to imposing, mushroom-headed figures.[13]

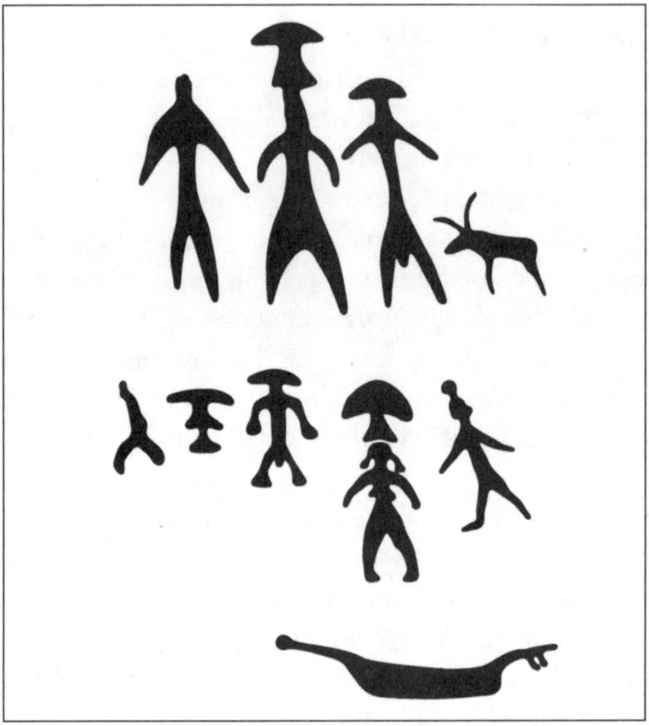

In 1967, archaeologist Nikolai Nikolaevich Dikov found the Pegtymel petroglyphs carved into cliffs about fifty kilometers from the East Siberian Sea. The panels show people, reindeer, moose, bears, and hunts on land and sea, even whale hunts. The mix points to artists from both the ancient Chukchi and the coastal Eskimos.[14]

Dikov and several mycologists identified these as fly agaric beings. In the drawings they never take part in the hunts. They stand apart, larger than anyone else, set in formal poses, often in the middle of the scene, sometimes holding a human by the hand. Many are clearly male or female, with the women drawn taller and in greater numbers. Dikov tied these figures to the use of mushrooms in ritual, and to shamanism, especially in the recurring images of "dancing Amanita people."

Want some more *mukhomor* fun? According to the German explorer Philip von Strahlenberg, the amanita mushrooms were so highly valued and so scarce that only the wealthy could afford to buy them from Russian and foreign traders. The poor had to wait. When the elites held mushroom feasts, the less fortunate lingered outside, watching for guests to step out to relieve themselves. Then they'd collect the urine in wooden bowls and drink it.[15]

Why? Because the psychoactive compounds in fly agaric, especially muscimol, pass through the body largely unchanged while the body filtered out the nastiness. Therefore, drinking the urine of folks who were eating fly agaric could produce a stronger effect than the original dose. Von Strahlenberg noted that people did this eagerly, chasing the fading spirit of the mushroom wherever they could find it. When wealthy drinkers were unavailable, peasants were said to drink the urine of reindeer that had eaten amanita. It is not clear how they obtained this bracing beverage.

The rules around cultivating *mukhomor* were even more whimsical. For example, practitioners recorded in the Soviet period said that consumers had to come to the mushroom with a good heart and anger drove it away and could bring trouble.

When you found a *mukhomor* in the wild, they said, you could not cut it with a knife, flip it over, tear out the mycelium, or take one that was too small. Instead, you had to sing with joy and pick it only when it was ready. You had to eat an odd number, so one would always be left, and you could not curse at it or speak harshly. In some villages, men and women could take them freely yet in others, women were forbidden from taking the mushrooms. One Koryak woman told a group of mycologists in 1994 that you couldn't eat an agaric that had been sliced at the base. Instead, the mukhomor had to be collected with their dirt or, said the villager, "If you eat this mushroom, you will be jumping on one leg."[16]

Afterward, you were told to sleep. Dreams in that state were studied for signs of what lay ahead, or for warnings. At times, the mushroom's spirits appeared in those dreams and told you not to come back.[17]

Meanwhile, back in Northern Europe, there is also some speculation that Viking warriors may have used amanita before battle to enter trancelike yet rage-filled states. These warriors, known for their ferocity, were thought to have "gone berserk" under the influence of some mind-altering substance, and while amanita seems possible, there is little evidence that the red-and-white speckled shroomie can send you into a rage. Other researchers suggest *Hyoscyamus niger* (henbane) or even an alcohol-fueled ritual that eschewed shroomies entirely could have been the culprit.[18]

The problem, writes Lechter, is that there is too little hard evidence of true psychedelic use, and some groups used one type of psychedelic and completely ignored mushrooms growing on nearby dung. One of the only verified examples of an early human dragging around mushrooms comes to us from Ötzi the Iceman.

"The 'Iceman'—the Neolithic man whose wounded body was preserved where it fell five thousand years ago in the snow-capped Tyrolean Alps along the present day Italian-Austrian border—was found to have been carrying pieces of fungus strung upon a leather strap. These were of *Fomes fomentarius*, a type of bracket fungus that grows out of trees in hard scallop-like shelves and has been used as tinder since prehistoric times (pieces of this fungus have been found by the hearths of Mesolithic settlements at Starr Carr in Yorkshire and Maglemose in Denmark)," writes Lechter. "[Along with] *Piptoporus betulinus*, the Birch polypore or razor-strop fungus, so called because it is excellent for honing the edge of a razor. For what purpose the Iceman had them is unclear (metal razors having yet to be invented in the Stone Age): They could have been used for tinder, medicine or magic, or have had some other symbolic significance that is unknown to us."[19]

Finally, there is Santa Claus. Some ethnographers and historians link fly agaric to pre-Christian winter solstice traditions in Northern Europe. Shamans dressed in red and white collected the mushrooms, often found under pine trees, and distributed them as gifts. He also came down chimneys because Shamans used a "smokehole" above the regular entrance to enter and exit their yurts.

Another thread points to Nordic myths about Odin. Around the winter solstice, Odin was said to ride through the sky, trailed by demons, in a sleigh pulled by his eight-legged horse. According to legend, the horse splashed red blood and white froth that fell to the ground and turned into amanita. While the current mythos is a bit far from that early demonology, we still picture Santa in red and white, and mushrooms factor in Christmas decorations around the world.

Again, however, we're faced with the precision of history. First, we realize that Father Christmas came to us in the early 1600s and became cemented in our minds by Clement Clarke Moore's "A Visit from St. Nicholas." Coca-Cola put him in his red and white outfit.

The idea that Santa was some kind of mushroom trickster began in the 1970s. It seems to start with Robert Graves, who mused about it in some speculations about hallucinogenic mushrooms. A writer named Rogan Taylor wrote about it in a *Sunday Times* piece in 1980,[20] and by the mid-1980s it was in the *New Scientist*.[21]

Ronald Hutton later took a hard look at the claim in his book *Shamans* and found a few holes.[22] Siberian shamans did not ride sleighs. They did not center their cosmologies on reindeer. They did not dress in red-and-white costumes. They did not climb out of roof holes while in trance, because their journeys were not physical performances but inner ones. Hutton instead suggests that the prevalence of St. Nicholas in Shamanic tradition came when Christians tried to convert Siberian tribes, like the Khants, to their religion. The two belief systems began to overlap, wrote Hutton, and "the Khants were likewise observed sometimes to be offering blood sacrifices to St. Nicholas along with traditional gods."[23]

All these tales, from berserker Vikings to Santa Claus dropping mushrooms down chimneys to villagers drinking bowls of mushroom pee, formed a corpus of folklore that inspired many mushroom fans like Guercken to nibble, if not outright feast, on countless mushrooms that may or may not have looked psychedelic. Once you see mushroom imagery in history it's hard to miss it popping up repeatedly, like some kind of memetic fungus. It's also important to share these stories because modern mushroom lore is a mixture of woo-woo and genetic research. The tales of Golden Teacher (a type of mushroom we'll visit soon) being bestowed upon humankind by a benevolent tree spirit are definitely fun but, until the 1950s, most psychedelic mushrooms were simply considered a dangerous addition to any balanced breakfast.

Back to the banker. In the early 1950s, R. Gordon Wasson received correspondence that drew him deep into living mushroom traditions. One letter came from Blas Pablo Reko, a Mexican ethnobotanist who had long written about Mesoamerican mushroom stones and ritual use. Another came from Eunice Pike, a missionary and linguist working in Oaxaca, who confirmed that the Mazatec people still used psychoactive mushrooms in healing and divinatory ceremonies. Pike explained that the mushrooms were treated as sentient beings, believed to speak through *curanderos*, revealing the causes of illness, diagnoses, and other hidden information. For Wasson, this was evidence that mushroom use was not a relic of the past but an active religious practice.

Intrigued, Wasson wanted to witness the ceremonies himself. In the summer of 1953, during the rainy mushroom season, he traveled to Mexico with his wife. Reko had died by then, but the linguist Robert J. Weitlaner assisted as guide and translator on the journey to the remote town of Huautla de Jiménez. Travel required cars and pack animals along steep mountain trails, and the villagers were wary of outsiders. No one would talk to him. After days of limited progress, Wasson learned that a local, Aurelio Carreras, was a *curandero*. Carreras later conducted a *velada* that Wasson observed but did not join. During the ceremony, Carreras consumed the mushrooms and entered a trance, offering divinatory statements about Wasson's absent family members. Wasson later reported that some of these details appeared to align with facts he verified after returning home, including the fact that his son was not in Boston but New York in a "state of emotional turmoil."

"On returning home, however, Wasson found things to be exactly as predicted: The enterprising Peter had made use of his father's absence to hold a party in their New York apartment, and was indeed in a state of adolescent turmoil, having been spurned by his girlfriend," Letcher wrote.[24]

Although anecdotal and unverifiable, the experience reinforced Wasson's belief that he was encountering something special. These early observations informed his subsequent fieldwork, including his later participation in Mazatec ceremonies, and set the stage for the *Life* magazine article that would introduce sacred mushrooms to a global audience

The article, called "Seeking the Magic Mushroom," completely changed the direction of psychedelic research and inspired countless men and women in gray flannel suits to turn on, tune in, and drop out. The story behind the article was equally wild.

His first experience convinced Wasson that these ceremonies were unlike anything described in Western psychiatry and that their purpose was healing rather than inducing madness. Two years later, in 1955, the Wassons returned to the Mixeteco mountains. This time, they met Maria Sabina, whom he called Eva Mendez in his article. Sabina was a Mazatec *curandera*, and Robert Gordon Wasson became the first outsider to take part in a traditional mushroom *velada*. The experience altered his view permanently, setting the stage for a popular movement that would ignite Western interest in psychedelic mushrooms.

The premise for the 1955 article was simple: Wasson and photographer Allan Richardson (whose wife didn't want him to take any mushrooms) arrived in a remote Mixteca village. There, unsure as to where to go, they found the small city hall and met Filemón, a local official who, thanks to Wasson's correct pronunciation of the Mixeteco name for the mushrooms, *'nti sheeto*, accepted the men as true seekers. Filemón, it was agreed, would take Wasson and Richardson to meet a local *sabia*, or wise woman, Maria Sabina.

That afternoon, Filemón led them down a ravine to gather fresh mushrooms, which Maria and her daughter praised for their firmness and abundance. They agreed to serve them that night.

"Richardson and I were the first white men in recorded history to eat the divine mushrooms, which for centuries have been a secret of certain Indian peoples living far from the great world in southern Mexico," wrote Wasson in the introduction to his story.[25] Whether or not this was true is obviously impossible to tell, but this article, produced in lurid color on the pages of one of the biggest magazines in America, was certainly the first time many Americans had ever seen a mushroom ceremony.

Around 8:00 p.m., wrote Wasson, about twenty villagers gathered in a small adobe room. At 10:30, Maria cleaned the mushrooms, passed them through incense smoke, and counted out doses: thirteen for herself, six for Wasson, six for Richardson. Both men ate the shrooms slowly over half an hour. The taste was acrid, they reported, and the smell rancid.

By midnight, visions began: geometric motifs, palaces studded with stones, mythic beasts, landscapes of mountains and caravans. In a later session, Wasson saw river estuaries under pastel light and a solitary, enigmatic woman in woven garments. Throughout the night, Maria and her daughter chanted, sang in Mixeteco, clapped rhythmically, and delivered oracular pronouncements in the voice of the mushrooms. Wasson wrote breathless prose about the experience, essentially describing the first recorded modern mushroom experience:

> Before midnight the Señora broke a flower from the bouquet on the altar and used it to snuff out the flame of the only candle that was still burning. We were left in darkness and in darkness we remained until dawn. For a half hour we waited in silence. Allan felt cold and wrapped himself in a blanket. A few minutes later he leaned over and whispered, "Gordon, I am seeing things!" I told him not to worry, I was too. The visions had started. They reached a plateau of intensity deep in the night, and they continued at that level until about 4 o'clock.

"There I was, poised in space, a disembodied eye, invisible, incorporeal, seeing but not seen," he wrote, offering us the first written permutation of "Whoa, dude, trippy" in human history.

On a later trip, Wasson brought his wife and daughter, who also took mushrooms and described vivid visions. He witnessed multiple *veladas*, learned that mushrooms were used to diagnose illness, locate stolen property, and report on distant relatives, and confirmed at least four active species by consuming them himself. During many of these trips he visited Maria Sabina, and her village, for better or worse, became the new locus for psychedelic research.

Interestingly, Wasson received funding for some of these trips from an unusual source: the CIA. In 1955, Wasson received a letter from James Moore, a chemist at Parke, Davies, and Company. Moore explained that he had funding from the Geschickter Fund for Medical Research, which agreed to underwrite the 1956 trip to the tune of about $2,000. The CIA reported that Wasson was "unwitting" and had no idea that Moore was researching psilocybin for project MK-ULTRA, the secret government project focused on finding truth serums and other mind-bending drugs for a Cold War fought mostly in the minds of countless spies and politicians. This odd collaboration didn't come to light until 1977, when John D. Marks requested MK-ULTRA files through a Freedom of Information Act request.[26]

Here we'll take a moment to talk about the woman who truly defined the modern psychedelic movement, Wasson's guide, María Sabina Magdalena García. She was a shaman and poet who had never left the town of Huautla de Jiménez in Oaxaca, Mexico. Sabina was an expert in *Psilocybe caerulescens*, known locally as Landslides or Derrumbe. These mushrooms, believed to be among those used by the ancient Aztecs in ritual, held deep spiritual significance for the Mazatec people.

Derrumbe tend to grow in tight clusters, though solitary specimens do appear. They fruit from June to October, usually in disturbed ground where few other plants grow. The mushroom favors open, sunny spots with muddy, orange-brown soil and woody debris. It was first described in 1923 near Montgomery, Alabama, where it was found on sugarcane mulch, and now grows freely in parts of northern

Georgia. To María Sabina, though, these mushrooms were not just plants, they were people.

Born in the late nineteenth century to campesino parents, Sabina lost her father when she was just three. She was raised by her maternal grandparents and inherited a lineage of spiritual healers on her father's side, who used mushrooms to speak with God. She explored the practices of *curanderismo*, a healing tradition that blended multiple systems of belief, but came to see her role as that of a *sabia*, a wise woman whose work was more than physical healing.

To Sabina, the mushrooms were not drugs but entities. She never saw them as something to be taken recreationally or casually. They were sacred tools used to find what could not be seen.

Her *veladas* were ceremonies of language as much as vision. In trance, she channeled the voices of the "saint children," the mushrooms, through improvised chants and poetry. These verses blended Christian imagery with pre-Columbian symbolism, continuing a long tradition of indigenous spiritual expression.

After Wasson's *Life* article revealed details of her ceremonies, visitors from across Mexico and abroad sought her guidance. Some came in genuine need; others came from curiosity. The influx changed Huautla and broke the secrecy that had protected Mazatec ritual. Sabina continued to hold *veladas* into her later years, even using psilocybin tablets when mushrooms were out of season.

She later said, "Before Wasson, nobody took the mushrooms only to find God. They were always taken to cure the sick." She regretted what had happened, but also believed it was destined: "The mushrooms speak. They have always spoken. They speak through me."[27]

While Wasson never named her directly in the article, the clues were enough for seekers to find her. Rumors swirled that rock stars like Bob Dylan and Keith Richards visited her, though there's no photographic evidence. More certain is that Wasson's story turned Huautla into a destination for outsiders eager to try the mushrooms.

The consequences for María Sabina were harsh. Many in her community saw her cooperation with foreigners as a betrayal. They burned her house and murdered her son in town. She was ostracized, and she believed the mushrooms "lost their power" when misused by tourists and hippies. It was a sad tale of gentrification and cultural appropriation by a well-meaning white banker.

The article marked the beginning of the psychedelic era in the West and revealed the ethical tensions in such exchanges. Wasson approached the mushrooms with reverence, but his article fed a global appetite unprepared for their spiritual weight. Sabina and Wasson were cast as prophets for a new age.

María Sabina died in 1985 in poverty and declining health. In Huautla, she is remembered as both a sacred figure and a symbol of Mazatec identity. Her image appears in local art, her chants are preserved in books and recordings, and her *veladas* survive today as a living thread of an ancient tradition.

Wasson went on to speak and write about mushrooms as much as he could, all while holding down his job as a public relations person for banks. His contribution to the study of mushrooms focused on the new concepts of ethnomycology, the idea that mushrooms had a profound cultural effect on humanity over the years.

As he and Valentina collected mushroom stories, Wasson began to talk about the divide between enlightened societies like Mexico, Russia, Greece, and the Nordics, and mushroom haters like his fellow Americans. Andy Letcher wrote that Wasson and his wife "coined the terms mycophilic, or mushroom-loving, and mycophobic, or mushroom-hating, and separated the nations of the world accordingly, placing Russia, for example, in the former category, and Britain in the latter. Soon they had divided up the countries of Europe according to this strange dialectical axis."[28]

Most importantly, however, he began to write what amounts to the first trip reports. For example, he shared one such report in his little book called *The Road to Eleusis*:[29]

> As your body lies there in its sleeping bag, your soul is free, loses all sense of time, alert as it never was before, living an

> eternity in a night, seeing infinity in a grain of sand. What you have seen and heard is cut as with a burin in your memory, never to be effaced. At last you know what the ineffable is, and what ecstasy means. Ecstasy! . . . In common parlance, among the many who have not experienced ecstasy, ecstasy is fun, and I am frequently asked why I do not reach for mushrooms every night. But ecstasy is not fun. Your very soul is seized and shaken until it tingles. After all, who will choose to feel undiluted awe, or to float through that door yonder into the Divine Presence? The unknowing vulgar abuse the word, and we must recapture its full and terrifying sense. . . . A few hours later, the next morning, you are fit to go to work. But how unimportant work seems to you, by comparison with the portentous happenings of that night!

Public awareness, however, remained minimal until the 1960s, when LSD escaped the lab and entered countercultural use. At that point, the world's reaction shifted sharply with fascination and mass experimentation on one side, alarm and prohibition on the other. This eventually led to psychedelic criminalization in most countries by the early 1970s.

Wasson came to see mushrooms not as mere intoxicants, but as bearers of ancient wisdom. He believed that these fungi connected participants with a primordial, perhaps divine, realm. His writings helped launch the modern psychedelic movement, influencing everyone from Aldous Huxley to Timothy Leary.

In fact, Wasson was one of the progenitors of the Stoned Ape theory, the idea that early man spent his time munching on shrooms and discovering their prefrontal cortex. He wrote:

> As man emerged from his brutish past, thousands of years ago, there was a stage in the evolution of his awareness when the discovery of a mushroom (or was it a higher plant?) with miraculous properties was a revelation to him, a veritable detonator

> to his soul, arousing in him sentiments of awe and reverence, and gentleness and love, to the highest pitch of which mankind is capable, all those sentiments and virtues that mankind has ever since regarded as the highest attribute of his kind.[30]

Wasson's *Life* magazine article introduced the Western public not only to the cultural significance of sacred mushrooms but also to the idea that these substances could facilitate meaningful, even mystical, experiences. In doing so, the Wassons and Maria Sabina helped catalyze a shift in psychedelic research from models of illness to models of consciousness expansion and healing.

Before Wasson's journey, the Western scientific community's relationship with psychedelics was cautious and clinical. Researchers in pharmaceutical companies and psychiatric institutions had begun to experiment with LSD and psilocybin, but their approach was limited and, frankly, unsettling. Psychedelics were primarily viewed as tools to simulate mental illness, what Stanislav Grof later described as "psychotomimetic" substances, used to replicate psychosis in healthy individuals so psychiatrists could better understand the inner worlds of their patients. This lens emphasized pathology over potential, casting altered states as aberrations rather than sources of insight.

Otherwise, psychedelics were simultaneously thrilling and scary.

The first steps toward acceptance came though Albert Hofmann, a pharmaceutical researcher at Sandoz in Switzerland, who first noted the psychotomimetic effects of LSD in 1943, over a decade before Wasson's visit. He reported taking a small amount of the substance and going on a bike ride. He wrote in his lovely book, *LSD: My Problem Child*:[31]

> We went by bicycle, no automobile being available because of wartime restrictions on their use. On the way home, my condition began to assume threatening forms. Everything in my field of vision wavered and was distorted as if seen in a curved mirror.

> I also had the sensation of being unable to move from the spot. Nevertheless, my assistant later told me that we had traveled very rapidly. Finally, we arrived at home safe and sound, and I was just barely capable of asking my companion to summon our family doctor and request milk from the neighbors.

The milk, he notes, was a very rational and clinical decision, something he was surprised to even be able to make. Through the ingestion of loads of dairy, he sought to reduce the "poisonous" effects of LSD, something that might give the current-day psychonaut a bit of the ick, akin to drinking a few liters of White Russian while already drunk. That said, he reportedly drank two liters of the white stuff and reported no ill effects.

Hofmann also isolated and synthesized the active compound in magic mushrooms: psilocybin. Hofmann had received a sample of dried *Psilocybe mexicana* mushrooms from Wasson, who had collected them during his expedition to Mexico.

Back in the lab, Hofmann and his team began the careful work of extraction, chromatography, and testing. He identified two key alkaloids: psilocybin and its metabolite, psilocin. Psilocybin, it turned out, was the more stable compound, but psilocin was the one directly responsible for the psychedelic effects. With this discovery, Sandoz produced a synthetic version and released it under the name Indocybin, marketing it to researchers and psychiatrists for use in experimental psychotherapy.

The synthesis marked a turning point. It moved psilocybin from the forest floor of Oaxaca into the fluorescent-lit world of pharmaceutical labs and academic studies. What had been a sacred plant medicine in Mexico became, almost overnight, a subject of Western medical research. For a brief window in the early 1960s, psilocybin was legal, respected, and widely studied. Then came the moral panic, the scheduling, the backlash. But Hofmann's work endures, his small, white Sandoz pills became the baseline for everything that followed in psychedelic science.

Over time, Hofmann's stories became whispered legends in the psychiatric community. Early psychiatric researchers saw LSD as a potential "microscope for the mind," offering unprecedented access to unconscious processes.

In the late 1940s and 1950s, the medical and academic worlds reacted enthusiastically, with research spreading from Switzerland to Europe and North America. Psychiatrists, neurologists, and therapists explored its use for understanding schizophrenia, treating alcoholism, and catalyzing psychotherapy. This early period was marked by optimism and a sense that a revolutionary tool for science and medicine had arrived.

The most important aspect of this work came in the form of addiction care. Clinicians observed that substances like LSD and psilocybin could, in the right conditions, interrupt compulsive drinking patterns and ease the mental grip of alcohol dependence. Early trials in the 1950s and 1960s hinted that these compounds could temporarily quiet the brain circuits driving craving, giving people a chance to reset deeply ingrained habits. While many of these studies were cut short by political pressures, the idea never entirely disappeared.

In recent years, modern clinical trials have picked up where those early researchers left off. One of the most significant came in 2022, when scientists at NYU Grossman School of Medicine conducted a double-blind, placebo-controlled study with ninety-three adults diagnosed with alcohol use disorder.[32] Participants were randomly assigned to receive either two high-dose psilocybin sessions or an active placebo (the antihistamine diphenhydramine, a.k.a. Benadryl, which in high doses, is a deliriant) alongside psychotherapy. Neither participants nor researchers knew who was in which group.

Over the eight months following the first treatment, the psilocybin group reduced their heavy drinking days by an average of 83 percent compared with baseline. The placebo group also improved, but by a smaller margin, about 51 percent. By the end of the study period, nearly half (48 percent) of the psilocybin group had stopped drinking entirely, compared with about one-quarter (24 percent) of the placebo group.

"Our findings strongly suggest that psilocybin therapy is a promising means of treating alcohol use disorder, a complex disease that has proven notoriously difficult to manage," said study author Michael P. Bogenschutz, MD, director of NYU Langone's Center for Psychedelic Medicine.[33]

This study built on decades-old observations, but with the benefit of modern safety protocols, psychotherapy integration, and rigorous statistical design. The results suggest that psilocybin's potential in treating alcoholism lies not just in dampening cravings but in catalyzing psychological insight, helping patients reframe their relationship with alcohol in ways that stick.

Valentina's appreciation of fly agaric has echoed well into the twenty-first century. Back in 2023 when I was first exploring the magic of mushrooms, I spoke with Psyched Wellness CEO Jeff Stevens about modern amanita mushrooms use.

First, he noted that amanita mushrooms have few legal restrictions in the United States, primarily because they can't be eaten without extensive processing. Unlike psilocybin, fly agaric was never scheduled as a drug. That legal gap allowed Stevens's team to spend two years working with KGK Sciences in Canada to produce scientific safety data reviewed by independent experts, before bringing their flagship tincture, Calm, to market.

Calm is a 30ml liquid extract designed to promote, well, calm. It comes in a small dropper bottle that looks like something out of a modern Wiccan apothecary. Its active compound, muscimol, is produced through an extraction process that converts toxic ibotenic acid into a safe, consumable form. Stevens calls it "CBD 2.0." It's not psychedelic but aimed at the same wellness space.

Stevens is a hale and hearty CEO with a full beard, going to gray. He spoke to me over Zoom and is much more a businessman than a psychonaut, spending twenty years in the capital markets while taking three companies public in a reverse takeover. He's essentially Wasson without the extensive travel and Siberian wife.

"There are no psychedelic properties, right?" I asked before taking the extract. "It's essentially more like a melatonin-style thing?"

"I would say that's a fair analogy. The way that we extracted and packaged it, the use for our product would be like CBD in the sense of 'Here's a natural compound from a fungus that, when extracted and used properly, it's going to have those benefits for you.'"

"And how do you get around the perception of *Amanita muscaria* being considered poisonous?"

"Well, that was the opportunity. My cofounder, David Chisel, and I started the company, and when he identified *Amanita muscaria,* I googled it and said, 'What are you talking about? This is a poisonous mushroom. You're crazy.'

"He said 'no, people have been consuming this for five thousand years,'" he said. "Siberian shamans have been using this for ceremonies, and there's a long history of use. So that prompted our first scientific studies to ensure that we could get a safe-for-human-consumption extract from this.

"I think one of the reasons this mushroom was never scheduled as a drug is that if you were to pick it like you would a psilocybin mushroom and eat it, you'd probably get quite sick. One of the compounds in it is called Ibotenic acid, and that's quite a nasty compound if it's not treated and can make you quite ill. So, the extraction process that we've designed converts the bulk of that Ibotenic acid into muscimol. The resulting extract that we have has been determined to have no Ibotenic acid. So, we end up with a muscimol extract, which has been deemed safe for human consumption. And again, it's a mushroom. It's food, never scheduled as a drug."

The mushroom cannot be cultivated in labs, growing only in symbiosis with birch and pine forests. The company sources it through a network of trained foragers in Eastern Europe, moving operations away from Russia and Ukraine due to the war. Sustainable picking ensures spore distribution and optimal compound retention.

Stevens is critical of the recreational market, where poor extraction practices, mislabeled products, and even psilocybin sold as amanita are common. He sees that as damaging to the category. His vision for amanita is as a wellness supplement, suited to dispensary shelves next to melatonin and CBD. Sleep, he notes, is the largest health category worldwide.

"Are you having any trouble with the push to legalization and the boom in illicit and potentially legal mushroom products?" I asked Stevens.

He frowned.

"Yeah, that's a different category for us," he said. "We're not trying to compete with the basement chemists. We're not trying to compete in the recreational space. We think, quite frankly, that amanita is not a recreational mushroom. If you take a larger dosage of it, you'll feel quite inebriated, and then you're going to pass out and have these crazy dreams, but it's not something that you would want for a party environment."

The tincture hits you about thirty minutes after taking it and makes you very sleepy. You also get some very light, very manageable hallucinations when your eyes are closed. Essentially the patterns behind your eyelids become more formulaic, sort of like fractals. Then you literally fall into a deep sleep, during which time I experienced some of the wildest dreams I've ever had.

In one dream I was trying to find Bob Dylan in a modern university library. During the dream, I invented a new word ("jeckelate," which means to come together as a group, presumably nonsexually) and saw Bob sitting in front of the library eating cotton candy. We talked quite a bit, and his commentary was at once banal and profound. The only thing I remember is how real it seemed and how wonderful it felt to be sitting with a childhood hero.

The fact that I could remember these details, including the newly coined word, was a first for me. I could see the value of these deep dreams in a population beset by cold, disease, and angry wild animals. Even lucidly dreaming about a sunny day thanks to these would be worth the price of admission, even it did consist of drinking some rich guy's pee.

Thankfully, Stevens said that his process didn't require any of that.

So, from Aztecs to berserkers to Santa Claus to modern start-ups, mushrooms have invaded our world in ways that many in government find dangerous or unsavory. Quite simply, however, it's clear that mushrooms are here and here to stay. Now, on to the next burning question: How do they work?

Why Do We Get High?

First, let's identify which mushrooms will make you happiest and which ones will hurt the most. *Psilocybe* mushrooms are also often indistinguishable from other mushrooms, including poisonous species. The resulting confusion could lead to an upset tummy or, worse, death. So, the only way to tell if they'll get you high is to correctly classify them.

There are a few ways to identify magic mushrooms. Traditionally, mycologists grouped mushrooms based on visible traits such as the stem, gills, and cap structure. However, this morphological or structural approach often grouped both psychedelic and non-psychedelic species under the same genus, *Psilocybe*.

DNA analysis in the early 2000s revealed that *Psilocybe*, as previously defined, contained two distinct lineages: one consisting of psychedelic species that exhibit a characteristic blue bruising reaction, and another of non-psychedelic, non-bluing species.

As a result, the psychedelic, bluing species were retained in the genus *Psilocybe*, which was reclassified under the family Hymenogastraceae. Non-psychedelic species were moved out of *Psilocybe*, often into the genus *Deconica*, which is part of the family Strophariaceae.

In a study led by Gastón Guzmán, researchers noted that the official "type species" of the genus *Psilocybe* was *Psilocybe montana*, a nonpsychoactive, non-bluing species.[1] That classification caused confusion, since the name *Psilocybe* is widely associated with hallucinogenic mushrooms. To resolve the mismatch, the type species was formally changed in 2010 to *Psilocybe semilanceata*, making it a relative to the Liberty Cap.

Further genetic research clarified the evolutionary relationships. The non-bluing, nonpsychoactive species remained in the original family Strophariaceae, consistent with earlier classifications based on microscopic traits like spore color and cap structure. Meanwhile, the bluing, psilocybin-containing *Psilocybe* species were reclassified into a separate family, Hymenogastraceae, where they unexpectedly share lineage with genera like *Galerina*, some of whose members are lethally poisonous.

One more twist: A lesser-known genus called *Melanotus* turned out, through genetic analysis, to be nested within the non-bluing species previously classified as *Psilocybe*. These mushrooms, along with other nonpsychoactive members of *Psilocybe*, were moved into a newly recognized genus: *Deconica*. This taxonomic reshuffling helped clarify which mushrooms contain mind-altering compounds and which do not, a crucial distinction for both science and foragers trying to safely identify fungi in the wild.

None of this will be on the test, but it's interesting to learn about shroomie taxonomy and genealogy.

You'll notice an important point there: Psychedelic mushrooms bruise blue. This means, quite simply, if you manhandle fresh, not dried, magic mushrooms, the skin and flesh turn a deep cobalt. This reaction, which we'll talk about in a second, is the easiest way to tell if you're dealing with a potential psychedelic mushroom. In fact, in the wild, you must see a bluing reaction before anything else, and you should avoid the mushroom if it doesn't bruise that color.

All you need to know? If it doesn't blue, don't chew. But even that can be misleading. Some mushrooms, like the culinary mushroom bolete, also bruise blue, which can be confusing to novice foragers.

So how do *Psilocybe* species, a.k.a. magic mushrooms, work? First, let's get some old myths out of the way. Mushrooms love to make networks, and we've already discussed the Wood Wide Web and other clever ways they interconnect in an environment. It is one of the topics fungi lovers love to discuss: how the mycelium network supposedly copies our nervous system and brain cells and how mycelium mirrors our own neural pathways in ways that are supposed to inspire awe and spiritual wonder. While that's a fun thought experiment, that mushrooms make new connections in our brain just like they make connections between chunks of dried dung, it's not quite true.

But then scientists were stumped again after finding that psilocybin is not limited to *Psilocybe*. Other genera, including *Inocybe*, *Gymnopilus*, and *Panaeolus*, also produce it. A team at Friedrich Schiller University Jena and the Leibniz-HKI recently confirmed that *Inocybe corydalina* uses a completely different set of enzymes to make the same molecule. None of the steps overlapped with the *Psilocybe* pathway. As lead researcher Dr. Tim Schäfer put it, it was "like looking at two different workshops, both ultimately delivering the same product."[2]

This is a clear case of convergent evolution, where unrelated organisms independently arrive at the same solution. It also leaves an open question: Why psilocybin? According to Dr. Dirk Hoffmeister, "Nature does nothing without reason. So there must be an advantage to both fiber cap mushrooms in the forest and Psilocybe species on manure or wood mulch producing this molecule—we just don't know what it is yet."

The practical impact is significant. By mapping this second genetic tool kit, scientists now have more options for producing psilocybin in bioreactors, which could support pharmaceutical research into its use for depression and other conditions. It also shows that psilocybin has appeared multiple times across the fungal kingdom, reinforcing the idea that this compound plays an important biological role we don't yet fully understand.

In short, the true story of mycelial networking is not that it mimics the human brain to make us feel mystical. It is that fungi, through their networks, quietly reshape and sustain entire ecosystems from the ground up and produce chemicals that are both helpful to themselves and the humans that eat them.

The thing that makes us high is the same thing that turns *Psilocybe* species blue. To find out what it was, I called up someone I found on social media and who turned out to be a genius in the realm of mycology, Dr. Fun Guy, a.k.a. Dr. Gordon Walker. He's about thirty-five, with a Colorado-bushy beard and twinkling eyes. He looks like a fun professor or, more precisely, the viral online professor who has suddenly become insanely popular thanks to his online following. He has three million fans, all of them drawn to his videos and photos of mushrooms in the wild.

He's also a renaissance man. He finished a BS in biochemistry from the University of California, Santa Cruz, and a PhD in biochemistry and molecular biology from the University of California, Davis. He also offers "discreet" consulting on winemaking. He worked at Opus One, a high-end wine company in Napa, and spent a year as a cellar hand at Pelican Ranch Winery. After all, he said, yeast is just another kind of fungus.

Walker is a mycologist and biochemist. He says he bonks mushrooms with his hand or walking stick for fun in the wild and his fans love him. He's also deeply thoughtful, allergic to all the spiritual hype around mushrooms, and very good at explaining the messy overlap between science and psychedelic experience. He's a man after my own heart. He's not a grifter. He doesn't sell mushroom gummies. He doesn't lead ceremonies. He doesn't tell people to take this kind of supplement to be more virile or alert or high. He writes books and looks at mushrooms in the woods. That's it.

Above all, he was genuine. I wanted him to explain mushrooms for dummies.

I asked him: "Why do these things even exist? Why do we take magic mushrooms and then see weird shapes or really enjoy EDM?"

He laughed.

"That is certainly a side effect of the psilocin molecule," he said.

From there, we went deep.

"If you talk about magic mushrooms in a mycology group, you'll get laughed at," he said. "You need to call them *Psilocybe*. That's the genus name. And the one everyone knows, Penis Envy, Albino, all that, that's *Psilocybe cubensis*."

The species name *cubensis* means "from Cuba," the type locality where Franklin Sumner Earle first described it in 1906 as *Stropharia cubensis*.[3] German-born mycologist Rolf Singer later moved it into *Psilocybe*, giving the modern binomial *Psilocybe cubensis*.[4] Two other names you sometimes see in old literature, *Naematoloma caerulescens* from Vietnam and *Stropharia cyanescens* from Florida, were later folded into *P. cubensis* as synonyms.

Cubes, as growers call them, are anything but Cuban-only. They are a dung-loving, warm-climate species now found across much of the tropics and subtropics, especially in cattle pastures after rains, with records from the Americas, Southeast Asia, and parts of Africa and Australasia. Their current range likely expanded alongside cattle ranching in the past few centuries.

Ecologically, *P. cubensis* fruits on bovine dung and well-manured soils, with caramel-colored to golden-brown caps that bruise blue where handled. It has become the best-known psilocybin mushroom largely because it is easy to cultivate indoors, which helped drive its global popularity in the late twentieth century. Many named "strains," Golden Teacher among them, are cultivated lines rather than formally recognized botanical varieties.

"Cubes appear around the world," said Walker. "There are hundreds of different species. They're all just *Psilocybe cubensis* and different iterations of the same thing in the same way that, you know, brassicas have been turned into kale and cabbage and what have you."

"There's a massive number of *Psilocybe* species that grow wild in nature. Typically, they are growing in wood chips, at least here on the West Coast. You're not going to see them really in the forest, which is funny because I get asked a lot: 'Like, where do I go to find magic mushrooms?' Just go to an apartment complex or some local park where there happens to be wood chips spread every year and some irrigation. And you tend to see these mushrooms pop up, you know, sometimes in huge amounts. You won't find them in the type of place you'd want to go on a mushroom hunting adventure, but in more of a place where you'd walk your dog."

"Why do they like wood chips?" I asked.

"They're wood lovers and they like to degrade wood. And some of it might be coming in on timber that we import. Over here we get nice wet conditions, and they come up in huge amounts."

Care must be taken, however. Many of the spots Walker describes could be sprayed with nasty chemicals designed to get rid of things like psychedelic mushrooms and other unexpected flora. While it's fun to dig through wood chips in the wild, the results could lead to an upset tummy or worse.

Many psychedelic mushrooms, especially those found growing near populated areas, are often lumped together, although they are distinct species. But several mycologists and growers argue they're likely just part of a broader species complex, genetically similar, with overlapping characteristics and the ability to hybridize. In practice, the differences between them often come down to specific strain histories and where they've been found or cultivated. They tend to thrive in similar environments, and many of them are quite potent. But someone, like Walker from the Pacific Northwest, might find one strain and cross it with another they know in order to create another called Walker's Strain or, more likely, Freaky-Headed Giant Purple People Eater or whatever whimsical name they can think of for a mushroom that can make you see God.

The strength of a mushroom's effects isn't solely determined by how much psilocybin it contains, said Walker. While psilocybin is the primary psychoactive compound, others like baeocystin, norbaeocystin, and aeruginascin may influence how it's felt. Psilocin is the active form of psilocybin in the human body, produced when psilocybin is broken down after ingestion. While psilocybin is more stable and typically the dominant compound in freshly harvested mushrooms, psilocin is also present in wild mushrooms, just in lower and more variable concentrations. It tends to degrade quickly when exposed to heat, oxygen, or light, which is why it's often less abundant in dried or older specimens.

These secondary compounds are chemically similar to psilocybin and may influence how it's metabolized or how it binds to serotonin receptors in the brain.

Walker compares this to the "entourage effect" observed in cannabis, where nonpsychoactive compounds like terpenes and minor cannabinoids modulate the overall experience of THC and CBD. In the case of mushrooms, the idea is that these additional tryptamines might subtly alter the onset, duration, or emotional tone of the trip, thereby making one strain feel euphoric and clear, while another feels heavy, introspective, or visually intense.

Though the precise pharmacology of these interactions isn't fully understood, early studies and user reports suggest that the unique cocktail of compounds in each strain may be responsible for the noticeable differences between varieties like Golden Teacher, Penis Envy, and Jedi Mind Fuck. In other words, it's not just the dose that matters, it's the mix.

Another quick aside: Walker also talked about *Psilocybe cyanescens* which means "turning blue," a nod to the vivid bruising. British mycologist Elsie Wakefield formally described the species in 1946 from material collected at Kew Gardens, giving it the modern name *Psilocybe cyanescens*.[5]

In the field, these mushrooms have caramel to chestnut-brown wavy caps when moist that fade to pale buff as they dry, with a distinctively wavy margin at maturity. They drop a dark purplish-brown spore print.

Ecologically, *P. cyanescens* is a wood lover. Today it fruits most often in urban and suburban mulch beds, on wood chips, and other lignin-rich debris, sometimes in dense patches. Its modern range centers on the Pacific Northwest and extends to the San Francisco Bay Area, Western and Central Europe, parts of West Asia, and New Zealand, likely spread in part by commercial wood chip supply chains.

Unlike dung-loving *P. cubensis*, wavy caps cue on cool, wet weather and typically appear in fall when temperatures drop. Because deadly lookalikes like *Galerina marginata* also grow on wood chips, careful identification is essential. Many foragers recommend going out with someone who is knowledgeable about the vagaries of various strains and who can tell different species apart. Even then, however, dangers persist. Even identification guides, traditionally a trusted source for mushroom lore, are being produced at an alarming clip using AI. These "guides" are messy, weird, and full of inaccuracies.

Culturally, *P. cyanescens* is well known among foragers and mycophiles, but it is considered harder to cultivate indoors than *P. cubensis*, which helped keep wavy caps more rooted in outdoor, wood-based habitats. The combination of strong blue bruising, wavy cap margin, and wood chip habitat has made this species emblematic of the "mulch mushroom" phenomenon in temperate cities.

So, from this we have the two primary types: *cubensis* and *cyanescens*. Almost all mushrooms fall into one of those categories, like the two types of cannabis, sativa and indica.

Now for the real question: Why do mushrooms contain psilocybin? Walker suspects it has something to do with a crossover from the viral world.

"A really interesting factoid that I have seen manifested in different ways is that psilocybin is part of a gene cluster. And I don't know if you've heard of the concept of Richard Dawkins's selfish gene. It's this idea that genes may have their own sort of desire to replicate," he said. "And this may come from the fact that some of these genes are actually old viruses that are integrated into a genome. And they may still want to jump around and move their genetic material selfishly, independent of the organism that they are part of as a larger whole. You see those with lots of different things bacteria and fungi do, you know, various sorts of jumping genes, transposons, things that go around. But psilocybin is in a lot of different genetic backgrounds. So, it's most common in *Psilocybe*."

"Outside of *Psilocybe*, there's a number of other saprotrophic fungi, including *Panaeolus*, *Gymnopilus*, *Pluteus*. There are members of these genera that are not entirely psychedelic but that have acquired this psilocybin gene cluster. And the question is, how did that transfer? It looked like some sort of lateral horizontal genetic transfer. And that's possibly because all these mushrooms grow in similar habitats. And so maybe their mycelium is smushed up against each other. And maybe there's a microvirus or some other kind of thing that facilitated the exchange of that genetic material. And then for some reason, it's been propagated and carried on. So, it must provide some sort of benefit. Otherwise, why would you carry this thing that costs energy to produce?"

Interestingly, Walker said, mushrooms might be using us to reproduce and spread. Mushrooms don't just grow in forests or on cow dung. They grow in our basements, in our grow rooms, and our barns. We use them in our rituals, our kitchens, our festivals, and our therapy rooms. We spread their spores for them, sending them out into the wild when we pick them and carry them around. And when you zoom out just a little, you start to see something strange: Fungi are shaping our world in ways we rarely notice. Not just through decomposition or soil building, but by shaping of our consciousness. Instead of just destroying wood chips, they're changing our culture. Name another living thing besides maybe a friendly dog or a good-looking apple that can get humans so excited.

Walker went on to talk about a concept in biology called the extended phenotype, also coined by Richard Dawkins. The idea is simple but powerful. Genes don't just express themselves inside the body of the organism, but they can also extend their influence into the environment. Think of a beaver. Its dam isn't part of its body, but it's still a direct result of its genes. The dam floods the surrounding area, creates a pond, reshapes ecosystems. That's part of the beaver's extended phenotype. Its genes are quite literally rewriting the landscape.

Fungi do this too, only in stranger ways. The extended phenotype of fungi is not always obvious. Take yeast, the simple single-celled fungus responsible for alcoholic fermentation. Yeast has traveled the globe with humans, riding in barrels, bottles, and bellies. It has fueled empires, sparked conflicts, built cities, and ruined lives. Wine, beer, and whiskey are all made possible by a fungus. In some cellars, house yeast populations persist for centuries and shape a distinctive style. Early brewers simply left their grain mash or crushed grapes exposed to the air, allowing wild yeast to settle and start fermentation. Yeast did not just survive. It thrived because we carried it, bred it, prized it, and built entire economies around what it makes.

Now look at psilocybin.

A single, metabolically expensive molecule, made by certain mushrooms for reasons we still don't fully understand, has given rise to a modern revival of psychedelic research, mental health therapies, spiritual exploration, subcultures, festivals, fashion lines, and biotech start-ups. This molecule, born from a quiet little mushroom in the dirt, has extended its reach into human minds and institutions. It's shaping how we talk about trauma, depression, addiction, and consciousness itself.

Just as heirloom vegetables look and taste different from their modern counterparts, early mushrooms probably had much less psilocybin and blued differently, thereby telling us that our ancient ancestors probably had a much harder time figuring out what to eat. But as we started picking and spreading the spores of high-psilocybin mushrooms, they became the standard for shroomies in the world.

Psilocybin isn't just a molecule inside a mushroom. Its influence reaches far beyond the cap and stem that produced it. Fungi, in this way, don't just grow in forests. They grow in language, in behavior, in global trade, in medicine, and in thought.

So, when we talk about mushrooms changing the world, it's not just a metaphor. They've been rewriting our script, sometimes literally, for thousands of years. And the stories they've started are still unfolding.

Back to the original question. From an evolutionary perspective, psychedelic mushrooms simply evolved to break down dead organic matter. They're saprotrophs, which means they digest carbon-rich waste, wood chips, dung, decaying leaves, and turn it into food. Unlike mycorrhizal fungi, *Psilocybe* species don't live in symbiosis with living trees (hence their love for wood chips and not mighty oaks). Species like *Psilocybe cubensis* are extremely flexible as to where they settle down, but this makes them unprotected by the sugars, water, and nutrients that trees provide their closest mushroom friends. Instead, they're built to take advantage of whatever decomposing material is available and to survive in situations that are considered harsh by these delicate mycelial networks. That adaptability, more than anything else, explains why they've stuck around and spread so widely. It also allowed mycologists to create a few theories as to why they turn blue and produce psilocybin.

First, there is the antioxidant theory.

As we said before, when you pick or handle *Psilocybe* mushrooms, the stems and caps can turn a dark blue. If you're not expecting it, it's quite jarring, simply because it's a blue rarely seen in nature. The bluing reaction is an oxidative process. "Some people think it helps the mushroom survive damage or stress," Walker said. "But again, that's mostly guesswork."

Another scientist I met, Ian Bollinger, offered to clear up some of that guesswork. In fact, he has some rather fascinating ideas about the source of psilocin. Psilocybin may not be the spiritual secret of the universe. It might just be sunscreen.

Bollinger is a biologist and data scientist with a rare combination of lab precision and programming fluency. He works at the intersection of molecular biology, fungal biotechnology, and automation, building everything from genomic pipelines to machine-learning models. With hands-on experience in clean-room environments and technical depth in coding languages like Python, Ian doesn't just run chemical and biological tests, he automates, analyzes, and translates them into structured datasets. His work spans everything from cleaning and merging genomic data to building image recognition tools and ML classifiers. In short: He codes, he cultures, and he connects the two in ways most researchers can't.

He's also surprisingly vivacious for a mushroom researcher. We spoke at length about his theory. With his jaunty glasses, shaved head, and fun scientist beard, it felt more like talking to a good buddy who just happened to know way too much about a specific topic than any kind of researcher.

When I asked Ian about why these mushrooms contain psilocybin in the first place, he laughed.

"Is it a happy accident?" I asked.

"Maybe?" he said.

He was careful to couch the discussion in the scientific particulars. He was a precise person and wanted to make sure I understood for all the talk of ancient rituals and cosmic healing, the molecule itself may have emerged not to enlighten us, but to protect a fungus from UV light.

Mushrooms don't make things unless they need to. Therefore, expecting mushrooms to produce a chemical that makes us high for our own personal edification or just for plain old fun is silly. Producing chemicals is expensive and takes energy. Therefore, Walker's theory that *Psilocybe* species were simply creating the chemical to keep us happy wasn't quite right. Like humans producing melanin to tan, mushrooms generate chemical defenses when stressed. Psilocybin, it turns out, is one step in a complex web of compounds. One of its cousins, psilocin, is reactive. When a mushroom bruises and turns blue, that's psilocin polymerizing. It forms a netlike structure that absorbs UV radiation, a kind of dye-based armor. As the mushroom grows and deals with outside stress, the bluing could keep it from drying out, ensure it isn't eaten by the wrong animal, and even protect the mushroom from harmful UV light.

In fact, the albino psilocybin mushroom varieties, which lack melanin, often have more psilocybin. Basically, the whitest mushrooms have to produce more psilocybin to survive, which is why they are the most potent.

Ian's research challenges a core assumption: that the genes responsible for psilocybin production determine how strong the mushroom is. They don't. Or at least, not in any reliable way. "We've tested mushrooms with identical psilocybin genes that vary fivefold in potency," he told me. "The genes are the same. It's the environment and the rest of the genome doing the work."

He compared it to the Y chromosome. It's associated with male sex traits but doesn't directly cause them. The real action is happening elsewhere, through a cascade of interacting systems. The same goes for mushrooms. The genes associated with psilocybin are necessary, but they're not the drivers of variation.

When the mushroom is damaged, cut, crushed, or handled roughly, psilocin is exposed to oxygen. This triggers an enzymatic oxidation process that converts psilocin into quinones and related compounds, which then polymerize into blue-colored pigments to protect the mushroom.

"When I get into the sun, if I'm lucky, my Mediterranean heritage kicks in and I end up with a nice olive tan," he said. "Melanin production is my response to UV. If we think about psilocybin mushrooms, or most mushrooms in general, they produce melanin as well to protect themselves against UV."

"That blue is a polymer of psilocin, very much akin to indigo," he said. "This is the backbone of a tryptamine, that six-membered ring and the five-membered ring structure. You can use that polymer from mushrooms to dye things, if you'd like. I've done it before. But that polymer is also UV absorbent."

"So, if a mushroom loses its ability to produce melanin but ramps up production of compounds like psilocybin and psilocin, which are already there because they might help deter herbivores, then that polymer, that chain or net of psilocin compounds, becomes a kind of UV protection. I'm not saying that's their only purpose—very few things in biology are exclusive—but it could be one way mushrooms compensate for the loss of melanin."

Instead, what affects potency might be how mushrooms respond to stress, UV exposure, insect threats, or even the nutrients in their substrate. These factors may nudge the metabolism into making more (or less) of these psychoactive compounds. The idea that potency is a simple matter of having a "strong gene" is just wrong.

This also complicates things for the psychedelic industry. If potency can't be predicted from DNA alone, you can't easily breed for it. You can't look at a genome and know what you'll get in the grow. And you can't patent the strongest mushroom just by isolating a gene.

Scientists have proposed that the bluing may also serve as a form of chemical defense, potentially deterring insects or microbes. However, the exact evolutionary role of this reaction is still under investigation. Bollinger's theory adds a compelling layer to the story.

There's another theory about mushrooms that seems even more interesting, especially given what another type of mushroom can do.

"The theory is that psilocybin is anti-herbivory," said Walker. "Like how plants produce bitter compounds to stop animals from eating them. The problem is psilocybin doesn't taste like anything. It kicks in hours later. That's a terrible deterrent."

Basically, scientists have long said that the psilocybin in mushrooms keeps birds and other animals from eating them. Or, more precisely, the mushrooms make psilocybin to encourage the animals that are affected by the chemical to eat and spread the spores. To understand this, we should remember another kind of fungus near and dear to the human heart and liver.

Out in the forest, animals don't need a brewery. Fruit falls from trees, yeast gets to work, and soon you've got a natural fermentation process happening right on the forest floor. Ethanol is just part of the ecosystem, a by-product. By filling up fruit with ethanol, the fruit and the yeast both serve their evolutionary goal of spreading throughout the land.

And this isn't just some light buzz. This isn't a Disney scene where a raccoon politely nibbles on a grape. We're talking real intoxication: dazed lemurs, wobbly elephants, birds flying sideways. The fermentation of sugar into alcohol is biology, not magic. And just like humans figured it out thousands of years ago, some animals learned the effects too, accidentally or otherwise.

Let's start with the African elephant. For decades, stories spread about elephants getting drunk off the fruit of the marula tree. These fruits fall, rot, and ferment under the sun. Locals claimed elephants would eat them in large amounts and end up stumbling around. Later studies questioned the alcohol content and how much you'd need to get such a large animal drunk. But more recent field observations and lab work suggest ethanol might still affect elephants, not because of volume, but because of how their bodies metabolize it. One study proposed that elephants have fewer alcohol dehydrogenase enzymes, proteins that help break down ethanol. That means even small amounts might hit harder.

Then there's the pen-tailed tree shrew. This little animal from Southeast Asia drinks nectar from the bertam palm, which ferments naturally and contains alcohol levels close to beer. But here's the twist: They do this almost nightly. And they don't seem drunk. Scientists think they've evolved to process the ethanol efficiently. This may be the closest thing in nature to a creature that can binge without consequences, essentially a wild teetotaler that drinks.

Even butterflies and moths have been caught feeding on fermented fruit juice. Some species rely on it as a sodium source. Others, like fruit flies, use it to choose mates; ethanol-rich environments can influence their reproductive behavior. In a lab setting, drunk male fruit flies tend to court less-attractive females. So, not much different from us in that regard.

Monkeys and apes, closer to us genetically, show more complex behavior. Chimps in West Africa use leaves like sponges to soak up fermented palm sap from tree hollows. It's not clear if they're chasing the buzz, but the ethanol is real. In fact, one theory, the "drunken monkey hypothesis," proposes that our ancestors evolved a preference for ethanol because ripe, energy-dense fruit often had traces of it. Following that smell led to more calories, which led to better survival. That could mean our own love of alcohol is evolutionary baggage. There, plants benefit because they are eaten at almost exactly the right time. A soggy, alcohol-filled fruit is great because it's easy to chew, the seeds are protected on the way down by soft fibers, and the drunk monkey is a bit more relaxed, so the seeds get spread just a little further through dung.

Ethanol, like psilocybin, has a very specific social effect. While elephants and moths might not be drinking to feel exactly what we're feeling, they are feeling something, and they're coming back for more almost constantly. The same could be said of these mushrooms growing wild in the woods. Instead of being anti-herbivory, the psilocybin is there to be eaten and enjoyed. Maybe, posits Walker, the mushrooms have the same effects on animals that they have on us. While the psilocybin might scare some of them away, it might give others a certain feeling or source of energy that is unique in nature. Maybe whatever animal or insect that eats a *Psilocybe* gets a bit of a buzz . . . or something even better?

But there's a bigger idea here, one that slips out sideways: Psilocybin might not have evolved for potency at all. It wasn't selected to blow your mind. It was just the compound that stuck around because it was a stable, useful, and convenient sunscreen. It could polymerize into a UV-blocking film. It could mimic serotonin well enough to confuse an insect nervous system. It could get stored in cells without breaking down. It's not the only molecule the mushroom could have made. It's just the one that worked.

And then, by chance, it happened to crack open human consciousness.

In all these cases, the substances in question aren't something separate from nature. They're a product of decay, fermentation, and opportunism. Animals aren't brewing in barrels or buying at dispensaries, but they're living in ecosystems where these things naturally collide. And they've adapted to it in different ways, some barely affected, others overwhelmed.

One fascinating theory[6] has been studied by researchers at the University of Utah. While some scientists believe that psilocybin is a deterrent like capsaicin, the chemical that makes things spicy, these researchers are trying to prove that mushrooms made psilocybin to keep slugs at bay.

First, we know that psilocybin looks enough like serotonin to click into 5-HT2A receptors, the same target most psychedelics hit. When that switch flips in mammals, insects, or spiders, behavior gets weird, although not as weird as what happens in humans as far as we can tell. Some argue that psilocybin acts as a laxative or emetic, helping spores pass through a gut before digestion, thereby allowing the mushrooms to spread far and wide while being carefully cradled in exactly the right environment they need for growth. So, perhaps the mushrooms developed psilocybin in the same way fruit trees developed the process of fermentation: to spread.

The idea, called the Gastropod Hypothesis, lines up the biology with Earth's worst day. Molecular clocks date *Psilocybe* to about 65 million years ago, right around the Cretaceous–Paleogene (K/Pg) boundary meteor impact that wiped out most life and left a world of rot. Fungi and land-dwelling slugs thrived in that setting. Slugs are heavy mushroom predators, and there were so many snails and slugs foraging that they overwhelmed biomes. If psilocybin evolved as a slug deterrent in that postimpact compost heap, the timing fits. The researchers are now testing to see if these mushrooms kept the slugs at bay.

Walker also said something that stuck with me. It was about the idea that organisms evolve in a myriad ways, and sometimes they coevolve.

I told him it sounded like the shroomies had a marketing department.

"There's an argument to be made," he said. "We pick them, carry them, grow them, talk about them. We spread the gene cluster."

That gene cluster, he told me, has jumped between species. Unlike bioluminescence, which follows a single lineage, psilocybin appears in totally unrelated mushroom genera: *Pluteus*, *Gymnopilus*, *Panaeolus*. "It's likely horizontal gene transfer," he said. "Some virus or mechanism allowed the DNA to hop between organisms. That suggests it offers some evolutionary benefit. We just don't know what it is yet."

Next, I wanted to address another theory, the idea of the Stoned Ape. It's the idea that humans evolved language because our ancestors tripped on the savannah.

Dr. Walker refused to go down the spiritual route with mushrooms. He has a very good reason: A molecule is a molecule, whether it gets us drunk, high, or sick. It has no spirituality.

"As a scientist, I get asked frequently about my spirituality. And I sort of usually try to respond with something to the effect of like: The more I understand about nature, and the deeper I dive into biochemistry, and the mechanism, and all this other stuff, it doesn't make things less magical to me. If anything, it makes it more magical, and almost more spiritual to physically understand what's happening," he said. "And then I still know that there is so much that we don't fully understand."

"And I think the most important thing about psilocybin is that it kind of holds a mirror up to ourselves. And I think everyone who looks in the mirror is going to see a different interpretation because it's shining through your own ego and self," he said.

Getting his explanation was helpful, and it's clear that there is plenty about the biology and history of mushrooms that will be helpful to us on our road to truly meet the shroomies. But the truth is that this molecule, as Dr. Walker calls it, has become a central part of many people's lives. From a rabbi in San Francisco to a sound healer in Brooklyn, from a CEO in Jamaica to a scientist in Denver, the mycelium network is expanding and connecting people who, just a few years ago, might have been too afraid to try mushrooms, let alone specialize in them.

We're arriving at this mushroom moment in 2026 for reasons that go far beyond novelty. The mental health crisis has pushed millions to the point where the old fixes, daily pills, years of talk therapy, and meditation apps are no longer enough. People are looking for something that can disrupt the cycle entirely, something that feels like a reset instead of a bandage. Psilocybin promises that possibility, and the shift is no longer happening in whispers. CEOs talk about microdosing in public. Veterans lobby for psychedelic access on Capitol Hill. Retirees join guided mushroom circles. Bryan Johnson, the guy who wants to live forever and has been giving himself blood transfusions and no end of ridiculous therapies, took five grams of mushrooms once a month for three months, a move that many noted would make him want to die. He described the trip as "exhilarating" and "positive," and said it dissolved his ego while simultaneously recommending it to seekers like him.[7] That he talked about all of this on X in the same way someone would recommend taking magnesium pills was the real novelty. What was once counterculture now rests in the same conversation as antidepressants and therapy, not as a replacement, but as another tool in the arsenal of mental health.

And unlike in the 1960s, the goal isn't escape. It's about engagement. People aren't trying to drop out; they're trying to tune in to their grief, their burnout, their buried trauma, their need for connection. That change in intention has opened the door for lawmakers, clinicians, and researchers to take psychedelics seriously. The politics are following the culture.

And that's what makes shroomies special: They're suddenly everywhere and they're helpful.

Golden Teacher

To truly understand mushrooms, I needed to grow them.

First, let me explain that I'm a consummate master-of-none-style idiot. I plunge into new things with the confidence of a white cis man who has never been called on his bullshit. This frustrates those around me to no end, primarily because many things require preparation and care, whereas I prefer to attempt new endeavors without thinking, resulting in failure. That I've been able to survive this long without electrocuting or poisoning myself is a testament to whatever dark god protects drunks and babies.

Coming from a home-brewing background, I assumed mushrooms would be as simple as beer. If you're a home brewer, you'll understand the ridiculousness of that statement. Home brewing is quite hard and requires a scientist's attention to detail and a doctor's preference for sterilization. I had neither. Sure, you can fake it, but good beer comes from a sterile, scientific hand and not a dilettante.

Sadly, years of product reviewing and journalism gave me the ego to think that I knew exactly what to do with only a limited amount of planning or even understanding. Whenever someone sent me something to review, a new phone or speaker or whatever, I immediately cracked open the box, turned it on, and hoped for the best. I never read instructions, which would have helped.

In fact, my wine- and beer-making skills should have been an indicator of my potential success with mushrooms. My wine, while drinkable, usually ended up in a sweet sangria or, given enough time on a Saturday morning, distilled into some of the foulest grappa you could imagine. My cooking style was nonchalant at best, and anything requiring precision, sterility, or patience wasn't my strong suit. I was better at assembling computers than cultivating mushrooms, and even there I was subpar, once coming in dead last in a timed PC building competition for charity. My PC didn't even turn on because I had burned out the memory chips by installing them backward.

All of this didn't bode well for my shroomies.

Before the carnage, however, I needed to answer a pressing question: Would I go to jail?

Without fail, the first thing my friends and loved ones asked me when I started this project was whether I liked federal prison.

Growing mushrooms is still illegal in most states, and while I won't say where I was growing, I wasn't about to make any friends at the DEA if I turned this into a business. Sadly, when it came to mushrooms, it was easy to gain that most desirable of economic factors: a surplus. That's the real problem with growing mushrooms: They grow like, well, mushrooms. During my research period, I produced so many so quickly that I had to throw some away and even skipped later flushes just to avoid having to find somewhere to put another massive batch of shroomies.

Even teaching others how to grow mushrooms is technically illegal. Since the 1960s, mushroom lore and instruction have circulated through books written by scientifically minded hippies. Terence and Dennis McKenna published the most influential growing manual in 1976, the *Psilocybin Magic Mushroom Grower's Guide*, under the pseudonyms O. T. Oss and O. N. Oeric, with, as the cover noted, "drawings by Kat and photography by Irimias the Obscure." The brothers, for their part, never explained the names. Some suggest they were a playful pun on *Stropharia cubensis*. Others read them as "Our Teacher Oss" and "Our Naturalist Oeric." The artistic style was part *Dungeons &*

Dragons, part *Anarchist Cookbook*, and it defined popular mycology for decades. This secret tome was hard to find, often tucked away in dark corners of head shops and crystal stores, and acolytes passed around copies like samizdat. Only with the rise of the internet did detailed guides become commonplace.

I soon learned that O. T. Oss and O. N. Oeric were right to hide their identities. In the United States, the legal status of psychedelics has barely shifted at the federal level since 1971. The Controlled Substances Act placed LSD, psilocybin, and mescaline in Schedule I, the strictest category, defined as having "no accepted medical use" and a "high potential for abuse." That meant anyone who dared to inoculate a pasteurized substrate, keep it sterile, and maintain exact humidity and temperature to produce a nonaddictive compound that lasts six hours, delivers visions of elves and geometry, and even makes jazz sound good, was legally a criminal.

That classification has acted as a brake on science and therapy for over fifty years. Researchers must still navigate layers of DEA bureaucracy for even the simplest clinical trial. It was at events like the one I took part in where researchers would do most of their underground research. In the absence of formal trials, researchers would poll psychonauts at mushroom events and therapy sessions. Unfortunately, this didn't lead to a very broad cohort to study, something that held back research for decades. Because these mushroom retreats were often expensive and, well, full of the same type of people, they wouldn't haven't gotten the widest representation of humanity.

In my research, however, I found that mushrooms were slowly becoming a less visible target in the war on drugs. The last big federal bust of note that I could find happened in 2016 when a group of men, Vitali Yaromin, Nikita Medvedev, and Maksym Lyushnenko, were caught with two hundred pounds of magic mushrooms in their Sheepshead Bay, Brooklyn, grow house. The trio also had $30,000 in cash and more than three hundred gift cards. As expected, the DEA villainized the shrooms to a hyperbolic degree.[1]

"Man-made drugs are our worst enemy these days. Those using synthetic cannabinoids, Carfentanil, U-47700, or psychedelic mushrooms are playing Russian roulette," said DEA Special Agent in Charge James J. Hunt. Considering psychedelic mushrooms were far from man-made, the comparison is a bit disingenuous, especially considering they grow wild in New York State.

That case was apparently the last one prominently featured on the DEA's website, with psilocybin ranking far below synthetic drugs and fentanyl after about 2020. Now, New York has a few integration service providers and many ketamine clinics with psychologists who are, *wink wink*, also proficient in other forms of psychedelic therapy.

States and cities have begun to chart their own course. Oregon's Measure 109, passed in 2020, created the first regulated psilocybin services program. Adults can now access psilocybin at licensed centers under trained facilitators. This isn't a medical model but a supervised adult-use system. Colorado's Proposition 122, passed in 2022, went further by decriminalizing personal possession and cultivation while directing the state to license "healing centers." Lawmakers followed with SB23-290 in 2023 to flesh out the rules.

It took serious money to get there. For example, multiple lobbying organizations dropped large donations to obtain legislation that would make shroomies legal. One group, Natural Medicine Colorado, is an advocacy organization formed to support the decriminalization and regulated access of plant and fungal psychedelics. Another one, Citizens for Natural Medicine, is a campaign committee created to back specific ballot measures related to psychedelic reform. It functioned primarily as a fundraising and political vehicle, channeling donations into advertising, outreach, and voter mobilization. In turn, much of its financial support came from New Approach PAC, a national political action committee that has funded psychedelic reform efforts in multiple states and helped coordinate strategy across campaigns. The two groups, Natural Medicine Colorado and Citizens for Natural Medicine, raised about $5.8 million, with $4.6 million from the national New Approach PAC.

The pitch was straightforward: Psychedelics aren't addictive, and the evidence shows they can help with depression, anxiety, and end-of-life distress. Johns Hopkins, UCLA, and NYU studies support that view, and the FDA has even granted psilocybin "breakthrough therapy" status for treatment-resistant depression. It was official recognition that it worked where other methods failed.

This state-level movement marks a sharp break from the 1970s and 1980s, when prohibition was absolute. As Andy Letcher notes, mushrooms went underground for decades, surviving in small circles of "hippies, freaks, and travelers,"[2] until cultural winds shifted and European loopholes briefly allowed retail sales in the 1990s and 2000s. Now, at least in my anecdotal research, the average psychedelic user is older, richer, and more hygienic than any 1960s psychonaut. One event I attended featured former hippies turned grandparents who remembered their first gritty trips with horror but loved blissing out to acoustic guitar on a yoga mat.

Complete societal acceptance of psychedelics is coming quickly. Recently I saw Colorado State Governor Jared Polis at a major psychedelics conference in 2025, where he essentially pardoned all street-level convictions for psilocybin or psilocin.

"Colorado has been a national leader in breaking through outdated laws around cannabis, and now we are doing the same for natural medicine," he told a packed hall in Denver at an event I attended. "This action eliminates past state-level convictions for psilocybin and psilocin possession that would be legal today. With these pardons, we are fulfilling the will of Colorado voters, moving away from ineffective drug policy, and encouraging local municipalities to follow suit."

Polis went further, noting that Colorado had "truly acknowledged the error in public policy that led to their conviction," placing the onus on local police for enforcing laws that made little sense.

"We continue to move Colorado and the industry forward," he said. "That includes looking at regulating additional natural medicines like mescaline, DMT, and ibogaine. We are analyzing the potential benefits and risks. Of course, we want to recognize the risks associated with these medicines, but we also know there can be greater risks with less regulated overseas facilities."

The biggest issue enforcement agencies have with mushrooms is that they're so easy to grow. Cannabis is close, but mushrooms require far less effort. Many strains will even pop up in the wild if left alone. Michael Pollan, who wrote one of the first popular accounts of inadvertent drug cultivation in his Harper's story, "Opium, Made Easy," captured these difficulties with a wry sense of humor. His piece followed a "tall, breathtaking poppy, with silky scarlet petals and a black heart," a garden plant that, when nicked with a razor, turned into an illegal drug.

"Let me offer a friendly warning to any gardeners who might wish to continue growing this spectacular annual: The less you know about it, the better off you are," he wrote. "Because whether or not the opium poppies in your garden are illicit depends not on what you do, or even intend to do with them, but very simply on what you know about them. Hence my warning: if you have any desire to grow opium poppies, you would be wise to stop reading right now."[3]

As for me, what I was doing was technically legal until the spores turned into living mushrooms. Pollan noted that as soon as you knowingly ground up the pods or processed the sap, you crossed the line into illegality. The same holds for mushrooms. Owning spores and substrate was legal. Acting on them was not.

With that question out of the way, it was time to grow the shroomies. To begin, I went where all modern shamans go in search of esoteric truths and mysterious formulas: Reddit.

Mushrooms grow through a process I think of as making dirt cheese. Like cheese, you take something nearly liquid and coax it into something solid, so solid you can fry a portobello like a steak or even make leather from its fibers. Or, in the case of *Psilocybe* mushrooms, crunch down on a mouthful in a repurposed yoga studio.

But turning dirt into magic takes planning and care. The next choice was location: indoors or outdoors. Indoors means year-round production in a cool, dark spot like a basement, crawl space, or even a cabinet. Outdoors depends more on climate, patience, and a little extra care. Both are possible with psychedelic mushrooms, with more control available with indoor grows.

Not every mushroom grower wants to stay cooped up in a basement with jars and tubs, however. Long before indoor kits and laboratory sterility became the standard, people were finding ways to grow mushrooms in the open air. Outdoor cultivation is closer to how fungi live in the wild.

Outdoor growing takes longer, sometimes months, even years, but it can yield steady harvests for seasons to come. You can mix spawn into compost, tuck it into damp straw in a shaded garden bed, or drill holes into logs and inoculate them, which works especially well for shiitakes and oysters if not some *Psilocybe* mushrooms. The main requirement is moisture. Mushrooms thrive in cool, damp conditions, and you may need to water often if your climate is dry.

Terence and Dennis McKenna noted back in the 1970s that psychedelics could fruit outdoors on compost if the local climate stayed warm enough through the growing season.[4] Unlike a small indoor jar, though, compost cultivation meant hauling in manure, turning piles, and tending beds exposed to the elements. It was less secretive and more like farming. That said, having someone identify your grow on a pile of table scraps and horse poop might be a tall order unless your local sheriff had done their research.

The Psilocybin Mushroom Handbook by L. G. Nicholas and Kerry Ogame later described a more approachable version: inoculating beds of straw, wood chips, or mulch with liquid mushroom spores.[5] This "patch method" works especially well for species adapted to woody debris, like *Psilocybe cyanescens*, which thrives in those mulched urban flowerbeds across the Pacific Northwest. Once established, a healthy outdoor patch can keep producing flushes of mushrooms for years with minimal effort, almost like a perennial garden.

Outdoor growing also reconnects mushroom cultivation with its cultural roots. In many indigenous traditions, hallucinogenic fungi were never separated from their environment. Mazatec healers gathered Derrumbe mushrooms directly from the hillsides of Oaxaca. Siberian shamans plucked *Amanita muscaria* from beneath birch trees. The land itself was part of the ritual. Planting a mushroom bed outside echoes that relationship, reminding us that fungi are not just laboratory curiosities but living organisms shaped by soil, climate, and season.

Of course, outdoor cultivation comes with its own risks. Yields depend on weather, and competing molds and wild fungi may move into the patch. And unlike a sealed tub in a closet, an outdoor bed can't be hidden as easily. But for those who want to meet mushrooms on their own terms, under sky and rain, the outdoor method offers something indoor cultivation rarely does: surprise. The grower tends the mycelium but ultimately must wait on the rhythms of nature.

But, again, I didn't have the luxury of acres of wide-open farmland or a hearty birch tree. I had a basement. I didn't have much room to commune with nature. My backyard is postage stamp-size and aside from a very small compost pile, there is very little in the way of wide-open dirt or broken-down wood. I'd have to head indoors.

The first step was carving out a small space in my basement for what amounted to a mushroom factory: a plastic tub with holes in it. I prepared a little table that I used to use for winemaking. It was a butcher block on four sturdy legs that I believe we bought from Ikea years before, and it was stained with grape juice and yeast. The next step was to figure out the easiest way to grow. Online, I found countless variations of the same instruction, injecting spores into a substrate and keeping them healthy inside a plastic tub. So I bought that plastic tub and poked tiny holes in it with a pocketknife.

So far, so good on the legality front. I now just owned a holey tub. Then I ordered my ingredients: two bags of substrate and a set of spawn jars. I also got an aquarium tank heater to keep the shroomies warm and an LED light that was supposed to let me trick the mushrooms into thinking it was a warm summer morning. I also bought a mister from Ikea, something you'd spritz plants with. Finally, I bought some spores.

Spores are also freely available, in prints or liquid suspensions. The liquid usually comes in a large syringe meant for microscopy slides. Note that I selected spore syringes versus spore prints. I wasn't quite ready to produce my own solution or petri dish of mycelium.

In fact, spore prints, for many growers, mark the first step into real mycology as opposed to my hobbyist junk. To create a spore print, you place a mushroom cap, gills-down, on foil or paper, wait overnight, and a dusting of spores falls, leaving the ghost image of the gills. It is both a fingerprint and keepsake, unique to the species.

Spore prints are more than identification tools. They help distinguish lookalikes, supply researchers with raw material, and let cultivators store genetics. For hobbyists, a print is proof that you grew a mushroom. In the culture, it became a rite of passage, a sign you had moved from looking to studying, from spectator to participant.

Growing gear beyond a tub and some dirt can get expensive. Today, there is a renaissance in mushroom cultivation. Social feeds are full of robots and kits for budding mycologists that, again, *wink wink*, are designed for culinary use only. Those systems require substrate subscriptions and run on an app, which means you can put your spores into a grower, and they should, in theory, mature automatically without any hands-on effort. Much like bread makers of old, companies like Rye and their euphoniously named Smart Mushroom Grow Box sell one-stop shops for lazy mycologists.

Interestingly, these mushroom robots shouldn't be confused with research done by scientists at Cornell. In 2024, they unveiled robots powered not by silicon chips but by mushrooms. By integrating the mycelium of king oyster mushrooms into their hardware, the team built a wheeled bot and a soft-bodied star-shaped robot that both responded to environmental cues through the fungus's natural electrical signals.[6] When exposed to light, the fungal network altered the robots' movements, demonstrating that mycelium can act as both sensor and controller. They even made a creepy-looking Terminator robot with mushroom skin to imbue the thing with the sense of touch.

But many of these robotic products are too hard on our shroomies. Psychedelics are fragile, sickly, prone to infection, and far less forgiving than culinary varieties. True psychedelic suppliers are far more clinical and well-sanitized and usually don't depend on an expensive box that heats up and sprays water on some dirt. None of these companies want to be associated with psychedelics. Companies like North Spore offer instructional videos and detailed instructions for home growers but remind you, in small print, that "North Spore's products shall only be used for lawful purposes."

Back to my tub of spores.

I always knew what I wanted to grow first: Golden Teacher, the easiest mushroom, according to one dude on Reddit. It was also the first mushroom I ate, way back at that first, grumpy trip with my friend Greg. I didn't know what they looked like, they came to me in powder form, but I loved the name, another nod to the *Dungeons & Dragons* lover in me.

As we said before, growing mushrooms was frustrating, exacting, and capricious. Therefore, my first mushroom, the Golden Teacher, led to many valuable lessons in handling all those things. It was actually a pretty good teacher.

Golden Teacher, a *Psilocybe cubensis*, is one of the most recognizable psilocybin mushrooms in the world. If you've ever seen a psychedelic poster featuring badass skull heads and weird mushrooms, you've probably seen Golden Teacher. Its name comes from the golden hue of its wide, shimmering caps and from the reputation it has earned among growers and psychonauts as a kind of patient instructor. It's the mushroom we first talked about in the last chapter, the one discovered in Cuba but that probably traveled around the world to get there. *Cubensis* is a dung lover, so I figured I couldn't mess it up too badly because it was already growing in poop.

I was wrong.

I pulled up Paul Stamets's *Psilocybin Mushrooms of the World* and got engrossed for a bit. This book is a classic, featuring an endless cavalcade of genera complete with color photographs taken by Stamets himself. Stamets grew up in rural Ohio as a kid who preferred the woods to the classroom. He struggled with a stutter and as a teenager bought a bag of mushrooms and walked to a special tree at the top of a hill. The bag contained about twenty grams of shroomies, and because there were no books about mushrooms, he had no idea how to dose himself properly. As he climbed the tree, a decidedly dangerous thing to do on mushrooms, he began to see a summer storm boiling on the horizon.

"I grabbed the tree and held onto the tree," he said to Joe Rogan. "The atmosphere became liquid."[7]

He felt a "powerful spiritual cleanse" and then felt a deep fear during the lashing storm. While he held on, he told himself that he would stop stuttering if he survived the ordeal. He said it "dozens, hundreds of times, over and over and over."

And it worked. The next day he stopped stuttering completely, a testament to the odd effect shroomies have on our minds and how intention in any trip situation is key. In short, you must tell yourself (and the mushrooms) what you want, and they'll try to supply it.

This wild story defined Stamets's love of mycology and over time, mushrooms became both his refuge and his mission. Stamets went on to study mycology in earnest, though much of his education came outside formal institutions, through collecting, cultivating, and experimenting. So, I trusted this guy to know something about the Golden Teacher.

According to his book, the cap usually started out cone-shaped, sometimes with a little point in the middle, before flattening with age. Young mushrooms had a rich reddish-brown color that fades over time to golden, then pale yellow or even white at the edges, while the center stayed darker. When wet, the cap could look shiny or sticky, but it dried smooth.

Underneath, the gills began light but quickly darkened to a deep purplish gray and eventually almost black as the spores matured. The stem was tall and sturdy, often thickening toward the base. Around the middle of the stem, there was usually a white, skirtlike ring left behind when the veil tore as the mushroom grew. The Golden Teacher itself looked as basic as could be, like the ideal mushroom from a storybook. They had a jolly little head, a long stem, and grew directly from patties produced by cows, horses, buffalo, even elephants in warm, wet climates. They were found across the southeastern United States, Mexico, Central and South America, Southeast Asia, and parts of Australia. In the US South, May and June were prime months, though they could show up into winter. If you were growing them indoors, however, the growing season was infinite.

Potency varied a lot. Some studies found *cubensis* to be moderately strong, but chemical tests show a wide range, sometimes a four- to tenfold difference between mushrooms, even from the same patch. Indoor-grown *cubensis* tend to be stronger than wild ones, likely because they're shielded from sunlight and grown on richer food sources.

Cubensis has also become the most widely cultivated psychedelic mushroom. Since the 1970s, spore prints carried home from Mexico and South America have spread worldwide, giving rise to well-known strains like Amazonian, Ecuadorian, and Palenque. These strains all share the same basic look: a golden cap, blue bruising, and a ring on the stem, but they differ in size, color tones, and sometimes potency.

In terms of effects, Golden Teacher is thought to be less aggressive than some other *cubensis* varieties, like Penis Envy. The psilocybin content is still significant, but users often describe the experience as balanced, visual, and introspective without being overwhelming. Reports emphasize feelings of clarity, connection, and insight, which explains the "teacher" reputation. Trips can last anywhere from four to six hours, with a gentle onset, a peak of vivid colors and flowing patterns, and a tapering into reflective calm.

When I took it the first time, I saw lots of fractal imagery, both when my eyes were open and closed. Like most *Psilocybe* mushrooms, it also changed my perception of time, making two-minute songs seemingly last for hours. I also felt a certain kind of expansiveness which made the room I was in, a stuffy studio full of sweating people, into a huge, airy lodge with amazing, echoing acoustics. Writing about trips is obviously quite difficult, how many ways can you say, "I saw God and she told me to listen to Miles Davis again?" but I'll try to explain my experiences here as clinically as possible.

Not wanting to do anything simply when I could do it backward, my first growing effort was in small, pasteurized jelly jars that contained a specially designed substrate. This growing process, known as PF Tek, short for "Psilocybe Fanaticus Technique," is one of the earliest and most influential methods for cultivating mushrooms at home simply because it was one of the first techniques spread widely on the internet through forums and message boards. Created in the early 1990s by Robert McPherson, a.k.a. Psilocybe Fanaticus, it seemed quite simple and scientific and reduced the potential for shroomies to meet bad bacteria. His idea was to make mushroom growing accessible to beginners by replacing complicated lab equipment with basic household items.

Sadly, McPherson suffered for his art. Seattle police arrested PF and his partners, including his wife, Amanda, in February 2003 for selling mushroom spores by mail order, a business that netted him about $30,000 a month. As is befitting a very online mushroom spore producer, McPherson described his ordeal in a long post on a public website still hosted, years after his death, by a Seattle-based ISP. He wrote:

> So I open the door and there they were, several men dressed in black, with helmets, shields, assault rifles, the guy in front dropping the battering ram to the ground, and in big yellow letters on their uniforms–D.E.A. The next thing I heard was, "get on the floor, NOW"! As I complied, the voice screamed at me again, "get DOWN, put your hands behind your back"! I got down as fast as I could in the narrow space between me, the door, and thc forward-thrusting black uniforms, shields, and big guns. . . . The raid was a real bitch. It was like the end of the world had happened.

> As I lay there on the floor, the realization swept in, and I knew my life had just changed. But I couldn't believe it would be in such a violent way. I expected to eventually get into trouble selling magic shroom spores. I was getting really famous and selling almost three thousand syringes per month with all of the usual idiotic nonsense from the usual percentage of morons who order (boxes coming back–undeliverable). But I had no idea it would be a full-blown DEA raid with automatic weapons and a SWAT team. I thought I would just be visited by a couple of cop cars and agents with a search warrant, and I would make an end. But not this way; it was as if I was an armed terrorist, or I was a wanted rapist murderer, or that I was a suspect in some kind of cop-killing or armed bank robbery.[8]

McPherson managed to walk away with the minimum sentence, while two of his codefendants had their cases dismissed. The US attorney acknowledged that from the day of the raid McPherson had taken responsibility, telling agents he was the one in charge and not hiding anything. What the DEA found at his home was small by any measure, a rudimentary grow setup and 11.4 grams of dried mushrooms tossed in a wastebasket. Even agents described the operation as "minuscule." Still, any mushroom cultivation, no matter the scale, carried an automatic level 12 felony. By pleading guilty and accepting responsibility, McPherson dropped to a level 10, with two points off.

Probation officers argued otherwise. Because McPherson had created the PF Tek and was labeled the leader of the so-called "PF shroom gang," they sought to add four levels, which would have pushed him to level 16 and a sentencing range of twenty-one to twenty-seven months. His attorney successfully fought that attempt.

The greater threat, however, was trial. Prosecutors warned they could calculate the total mushroom yield from the more than 100,000 spore syringes McPherson had sold, framing it as a conspiracy case. They had evidence: He bought extensive ads in *High Times* magazine, he ran a popular website, and he held years of bank and tax records from his business. He also had boxes of syringes. The DEA was able to grow their own mushrooms in their own lab using his cultivation method. By their account, the PF Tek worked exactly as advertised, and the photographic evidence supplied in the case proved it. On top of that came a parade of unrelated cases tied loosely to his customers, hundreds of returned packages, and frightened people who received syringes they hadn't ordered and called the police. Federal surveillance had gone on for years, even including cameras at a Seattle post office. Fingerprints on syringes, mailers, and money orders piled up as evidence. The prosecutors had wanted to make an example out of McPherson. It didn't work, and his technique survived in the pages of *High Times* magazine and online. Basically, the courts found that selling syringes of spores wasn't a crime, even if he also gave instructions for growing mushrooms from them.

In the end, the Feds returned a substantial amount of money, allowed him to keep three houses, and gave back his Chevy S-10 pickup and his wife's Honda CRV. For McPherson, it was far from freedom, but it was also far from the worst outcome the government had threatened.

PF stayed out of the headlines for a few years after his arrest and then shuffled off into mycology legend. He died in November 2011 after teaching thousands how to grow mushrooms simply and easily at home.

The PF Tek process relies on a very forgiving substrate made of brown rice flour, vermiculite (a hydrated laminar mineral), and water, packed into half-pint glass jars. Each jar is topped with a layer of dry vermiculite, which acts as a natural barrier against contamination. The jars are sterilized by steaming for ninety minutes, which can cause the glassware to explode. You then inoculate them with spores via a syringe through a small hole in the lid. Over the next few weeks, white mycelium spreads through the substrate until the jars are fully colonized.

At that point, growers "birth" the cakes by removing them from the jars, rinsing and soaking them in water to rehydrate, and rolling them in vermiculite. The cakes are then placed in a simple fruiting chamber, the plastic tub. Within a week or two, mushrooms begin to pin and mature.

The genius of PF Tek is its accessibility. McPherson discovered that adding vermiculite created a light, airy substrate that resisted contamination because you weren't using poop, sterilized or otherwise. All of this encouraged mycelial growth, and the method was so reliable that he claimed mushrooms would "grow virtually by themselves."[9] It quickly spread through the underground community, earning McPherson a folk-hero status.

Interestingly, McPherson's early growing techniques have been refined by multiple practitioners, including Travis Tyler Fluck, who, legend has it, adds colloidal gold to his grows before sharing the mushrooms with terminal patients to ease their passage. PF himself went to court so the rest of us could have access to simple, reliable methods for cultivating mushrooms at home.

That history was in the back of my mind when I set up my own jar grow of Golden Teachers, using spores purchased from a Canadian supplier. The box arrived covered in bold disclaimers: "For Microscopy Use Only"—again, fooling no one. The syringes were oversized, like something meant for livestock, and inside was a cloudy liquid with specks suspended in it. It looked less like a clean scientific solution and more like something that had caught an infection. In a sense, mushrooms themselves are a kind of controlled infection, spreading invisibly until conditions are just right for them to burst into view.

The next step was sterility. Official instructions suggested wiping the needle with alcohol swabs before each use. A friend of mine, who had already tried and failed to grow mushrooms, insisted the real trick was to flame-sterilize the tip until it glowed red hot. I followed his advice, holding a lighter beneath the steel until it glowed, then watching a thin layer of soot collect on the surface. It looked dramatic, like something out of a field hospital, though probably not the best thing for my shroomies. Still, it felt safer than going in with a cold needle.

Once the tip cooled, I injected a little spore solution into each of the six jars. The liquid seeped into the mixture of seeds and sand, carrying millions of microscopic spores with it. I tucked the jars into a dark closet and waited. A week later, when I checked, I saw a faint fuzz beginning to spread, thin white threads that wrapped around rye berries like tree roots. These were the first hyphae, the filaments that branch out, meet, and fuse into the dense network called mycelium. This is the real organism, the hidden body of the fungus, steadily colonizing every pocket of food and moisture in the jar.

Patience was never my strong suit. Instead of leaving the jars alone, I kept pulling them out, turning them over, and holding them up to the light, hoping for an overnight explosion of white. The reality was slower and stranger. For nearly two weeks, little seemed to happen. Then, almost suddenly, faint white patches began to bloom across the glass, like frost spreading on a window. In some jars, the mycelium worked invisibly beneath the surface before erupting outward, pressing against the sides as if an alien life-form had woken up inside.

Convinced the jars were fully colonized (reader: they weren't), I rushed to the next step. I cracked them open and dumped the cakes into a plastic tub I had half-heartedly washed with hot water. I should have used alcohol, but impatience got the better of me. The dense pucks of substrate sat forlornly on the bottom while I sprayed them daily, waiting for some sudden bloom.

Indoor cultivation is tricky for exactly this reason: contamination. The substrate is rich in nutrients, which makes it perfect for mushrooms but equally perfect for mold and bacteria. It's the same principle as homemade yogurt or wine: too much sugar and yeast, and the wrong microbes quickly take over. Once a single contaminant spore finds its way into a sealed tub, there's nowhere else for it to go. It spreads fast, unchecked, and can choke out the mushrooms before they even fruit. A grow chamber becomes a battlefield, and if contamination gets the first strike, the mushrooms rarely win.

Outdoors, the equation is different. Mushrooms thrive in the open because nature is balanced. Soil, insects, air currents, and the endless turnover of organic matter all help keep threats in check. Competing microbes are diluted across the vastness of the forest floor. Airflow and shifting weather scatter spores, preventing one colony from overwhelming another. Mushrooms evolved for this setting, not for sealed bags in basements. What looks like an ideal indoor environment is fragile. A single infection can wipe out a crop, while outdoors the fungi enjoy the resilience of the whole ecosystem behind them.

That's one reason I turned to companies like North Spore in Maine. They approach mushroom cultivation the way a homebrew shop approaches beer, offering supplies hobbyists can't easily produce themselves. Their catalog runs from ready-to-inoculate substrate bags to larger systems designed for repeated use. A popular example is their Boomr Bin, a sturdy plastic container with air holes precut into the sides. With it, you can grow lion's mane, shiitake, or other gourmet mushrooms in just a few weeks with minimal effort. For beginners, it's as close to plug-and-play mushroom growing as it gets.

North Spore also provides what mushrooms crave most: dung. Not raw barnyard manure, but pasteurized dung. Pasteurization strips out harmful bacteria and pests while leaving the dense nutrients fungi feed on. It's the perfect compromise, nutrient-rich fuel for the mushrooms, minus the competing organisms that would normally win out indoors. What looks like ordinary dirt in the wild becomes a petri dish of problems in a sealed tub. Pasteurization tips the balance back toward the mushrooms, giving them a clean, fighting chance.

To get a deeper look into the mushroom-supply industry, I spoke with Matthew McInnis, cofounder of North Spore, on a hot Denver rooftop. He was calm and collected despite the heat, while I fumbled with my recorder. McInnis has a background in photography and the look of a field naturalist, scruffy beard, tattoo of mating dragonflies on his arm. He told me North Spore began by selling fresh mushrooms to Portland restaurants before expanding into cultivation gear.

"My cofounders brought all the lab knowledge that underpins mushroom cultivation," he said. "When we started, we were vertically integrated. We were doing our own lab and culture work, producing spawn for ourselves, because at that time there really wasn't an industry supporting small growers."

From there, the company moved into sterile products. "We started selling substrates, then lab supplies, and eventually full growing systems," he said. "Education was another big focus. Today there are dozens of online educators talking about cultivation, but when we were starting out, it was a dead zone."

McInnis wasn't exaggerating. Now, creators like Turnip Todd and Just Alex rack up millions of views with mushroom-growing tutorials, while North Spore puts out its own instructional videos tied to its products. Beyond substrates, they sell humidifiers calibrated to maintain the 80-plus percent humidity mushrooms need, small fans to provide oxygen, and even full-size tents to keep contaminants at bay. Between the dirt, the gear, and the guidance, North Spore and its competitors can outfit nearly anyone.

The pandemic was the tipping point. "The sterile substrate category really took off around the pandemic," McInnis said. "People wanted to grow mushrooms in monotubs, but they didn't want to be cooking horseshit in their ovens at home."

That moment of excitement turned into a rush. Around 2020, mushrooms were hailed as the "next big thing." Entrepreneurs flooded in, including veterans from the cannabis industry chasing the next boom. Dozens of substrate producers popped up nationwide. But by McInnis's account, the bubble deflated almost as quickly as it swelled.

"The story mirrors cannabis," he said. "There was a bubble in mushrooms right after. The truth is you don't need nearly as many mushrooms to meet demand as you do cannabis. Still, money poured in. Supply outpaced demand, prices collapsed, and companies scrambled. A lot of the big names from a few years ago are already gone."

Part of the collapse came down to the challenge of making sterile substrates at scale. "It's expensive and technically difficult," McInnis explained. "You need the right hydration levels, precise autoclave cycles, and careful pressurization. If any of those fluctuate, even slightly, sterilization fails. It's a process full of peaks and valleys and getting it right every time is harder than most people realize."

Psilocybe mushrooms love the same thing their enemies love: warm, wet, nutrient-rich places. A tub or bag is exactly that. It is a miniature rainforest with no predators, no wind, and plenty of sugar and nitrogen. That makes it perfect for mushrooms, and perfect for everything that wants to eat or outgrow them. Out in the world, airflow, microbes, insects, and soil chemistry keep the balance. Inside a sealed box, once the wrong thing lands, there is nowhere else for it to go.

What happens when a grow gets infected is simple. First, you see a color or texture that does not belong. Then the smell changes. Finally, the mushrooms stop. The invader either steals the food, burns through the oxygen, or releases chemicals that stall the mycelium. A project that looked fine on Monday can be unrecoverable by Friday. That is the danger. Indoor cultivation concentrates risk. A single stray spore can set the clock running.

Here are the usual suspects and how they tend to show up to the party. The first is a bacterial "wet spot," also called sour rot, which is one of the most common problems. It turns kernels or substrate slick and translucent, almost like cooked onions. The smell is unmistakable, sweet-sour, sometimes like dirty gym socks, and you might see small bubbles forming on the surface. When it appears, the mushroom mycelium nearby often looks weak and thinned out. Basically, your spawn bag began fermenting and killed the mushrooms.

Trichoderma, a.k.a. Trich, the notorious green contaminant, is another threat. It begins bright white and aggressive, racing across the surface. Then, once established, it sporulates into a vivid emerald or moss green. By the time you see that color, the mold has already released billions of spores and, worse, it digs down into the tub, creating a pocket of mold that is impossible to remove. It wins through speed, quickly overtaking a tub. There is some belief that you can cut out Trich infections without damaging your mushrooms, but I didn't find this to be the case. As you'll soon discover, this was only one of many things I discovered to be wrong.

Cobweb mold looks very different. It forms wispy, gray, feathery patches, like breath fogging on cold glass. Left unchecked, it can cover an entire surface in a single day. Growers sometimes mistake it for healthy mycelium until it suddenly consumes the whole jar or tub.

Aspergillus and penicillium species also make regular appearances. These molds show up as uneven blue-green or blue-gray powders, often clustering around edges, scars, or uncolonized patches. Their blotchy, watercolor-like look makes them easy to distinguish from the pure white of mushroom mycelium.

The "bread molds," Mucor and Rhizopus, form tall, fluffy gray tufts that quickly sprout black pinheads. They thrive in still, muggy corners, the same conditions that favor neglected bread in a plastic bag. Once established, they spread with surprising speed.

Lipstick mold, Neurospora, is striking but just as destructive. It creates pink to coral patches that spread in sheets across the substrate. It might look attractive at first, but it spells the end of a grow.

Yeasts present differently. Instead of fluff, they leave a wet sheen, tiny bubbles, and sometimes a faint fruity odor. They don't make fuzz; they make gloss. Their presence often hints at contamination carried in with the spore solution.

Finally, there's Pseudomonas, better known as "brown blotch." It shows up more often in button mushroom houses, but it's worth mentioning. The infection causes oily brown stains on mushroom caps, sometimes leaving pitted or slimy tissue in its wake.

Pests count as infections too. Fungus gnats lay eggs that hatch into tiny larvae, which tunnel through mycelium and carry microbes on their bodies. Mites ride in on unfiltered air or on gear and leave little pockmarks where they feed. You do not always see the insect first. You see the damage.

What do infections do, practically? Three things. They divert nutrients, so mushrooms never pin or stall mid-growth. They change the microclimate, eating oxygen and throwing off heat and acids that stress the host. And they weaponize chemistry, releasing enzymes and antibiotics that slow or dissolve neighboring cells. A tub that was white and lively begins to yellow at the edges, then turns patchy, then smells off. Pins stop swelling. Caps wrinkle. Stems hollow. At that point, the outcome is decided.

There is also the human side. Some molds release spores and compounds that irritate lungs and skin. If a block goes bright green or black, the safest move is to bag it, seal it, and take it outside. Do not shake it around. Do not sniff it. A failed grow is disappointing but should not become a health problem. Black mold is an actual danger, and to open a bag of it in your grow area is to simply encourage more infections over time.

All of this might sound like fungi are delicate things, but the opposite is true. The organism fights back. Mycelium is a living web that senses damage, reroutes growth, and walls off trouble. Hyphae can fuse into thicker cords that bypass a bad patch and keep foraging. Many species secrete their own antibiotics and phenolic compounds that suppress bacteria and rival molds. Some produce dense survival forms, like sclerotia, that hunker down through drought, cold, and microbial attack, then reboot when the coast is clear. Others throw rhizomorphs, ropelike strands that leap gaps and colonize fresh material before competitors can get there. In the soil, this tug-of-war rarely ends the species. It just reshapes the battlefield.

Indoors, the battlefield is smaller. That is why infections feel so final. There is no fresh edge to run to, no breeze to thin the spores, no beetle to carry the fight away. A monoculture in a plastic box has two futures. It fruits, or it feeds something else. Because it takes so long to spawn, infections can drive growers crazy. To see Trich hit a tub weeks into a grow is super frustrating.

You can read a grow's fate in its signs. Healthy colonization looks bright, even, and slightly matte. It creeps with purpose and thickens where food is richest. Stress shows up as stalled patches, glassy or overly glossy surfaces, sweaty yellow droplets that are often just metabolites, not urine, and a smell that shifts from "earthy" to "off." Collapse brings colors, powders, slime, and a smell you will not mistake the second time. Most mushrooms don't appear colorful when they grow, so a bright green or pink is a bad sign.

Shroomies aren't delicate little guys. Fungal cells are walled with chitin and carry ergosterol in their membranes. That gives them physical toughness. More important is their plasticity. Most cells in a mycelium can change jobs. They can become exploratory tips, transport highways, or the beginnings of a fruit. When a front gets poisoned or crowded, growth pivots elsewhere.

So, what is the point of this detour? It is to say that every flush you complete is a narrow win. The same chemistry that makes mushrooms possible also invites rivals, and indoors the odds are tighter. When a grow goes bad, it is not because fungi are weak. It is because the grower is. When it goes right, it is because the organism outran everything that wanted the same meal and, especially, outran the incompetence of its grower.

Sadly, my shroomies couldn't outrun my incompetence.

That first batch, my first batch in this wild adventure, was a dud.

I'm proud to say that my Golden Teacher failed for an interesting reason: Once I saw my pucks had stalled, I decided to bury them in substrate. Then, being a moron, I placed my UV lamp directly on the substrate itself, essentially dumping a bacteria-infected light fixture into my grow. See, I thought you needed to put the light closer to the mycelium.

A few days later I saw my first batch of Trich.

The green spread out across the face of the substrate like an oil slick. My mycelium had been trying to break out into the substrate, then the bugs invaded and the mushrooms died where the Trich lived. But I was still unsure whether I could simply cut around the bad parts, like you would some grocery store cheddar.

Confused, I posted a picture of my grow to the r/contamfam subreddit, a group dedicated to identifying and, in my case, making fun of growers whose shroomies had gone rogue. I included the picture of my lamp lying directly on the substrate.

"Is that your UV lamp?" asked one. "You dropped that thing right on the substrate? Moron."

"Dude," intoned another. "Kill it with fire."

"You are a idiot[sic]," said yet another. "Throw that bin away."

There you have it: my first grow ruined by my refusal to follow directions. I swore that I would try again and this time I would spend more money and time on making something appear in my little mycological microcosm.

How to Trip

Because I can't keep my mouth shut, I started telling friends and family about my mushroom experiences. Everyone I spoke to said the same thing: They had done mushrooms or LSD once or twice in college, but now, thanks to kids, mortgages, and all the other things modern humans stress about while the world seems to be going to pot, they hadn't touched them since. Still, they were curious.

Except my mother.

"You have to throw away this shit," she said, convinced I was one illegal spore print away from turning into a *Breaking Bad* character. Luckily, she didn't live nearby, and I rarely listened to her anyway.

Once I was a self-described mushroom expert, the questions started. One friend asked how much she should take for a standard trip and, thinking back to my first time, I told her something like two or three grams. I gave her a little baggie of caps and stems, weighed on a digital scale I had bought for the express purpose of looking cool while parceling out shroomies.

"Ah yes," I said, trying to sound wise. "This is exactly eight grams. Split this dose in half with your boyfriend, or whoever."

It was not exactly eight grams. It was more like 8.25 or something.

"Can I pay you?" she asked.

"No way," I said. "I just want to get rid of it."

A few months later, I got a notification on my phone. My dried shroomies had failed. It felt like getting a disciplinary note from my kids' school. My little friends were underperforming.

"They didn't work," she wrote in a text. "I didn't feel anything."

I asked her the usual questions. Are you on antidepressants? Where were you? What did you eat? She had all the right answers: no, at home, and nothing.

Some trips stall or never quite take off. One friend was on SSRIs and found the whole thing muted, a trip he barely felt. Other friends, as we will see, would take a single gram and end up talking to the Old Gods of the Forest while wandering around a Target. It depended on the person, the strain, and the dose. Mostly, it depended on the person.

I told her to regroup and gave her a new baggie of mushrooms I had grown after those aborted Golden Teachers. She took four grams and later told me she had a massive trip.

"My body fell into separate parts and I was flat on the bed," she said. "I kept talking to my friend who I was with, asking for help, and he was equally helpless. 'I need to have my session,' he kept saying. So, I decided to make friends with things around the room, including my favorite plant and the ceiling fan. After all, it had five big arms that could hug me."

These kinds of reports were common. Everyone reacts differently to mushrooms, and no two trips are the same. When I spoke with a facilitator last year, they told me I should increase my dose if I wanted a specific effect. Taking the same amount each time was like taking the well-worn path home; you never see the place where the road diverged in the yellow wood and made you experience ego death.

Taking all this into account, what does the average mushroom trip feel like, and how do you go on one? This is the question most first-timers circle around. Let's get a little clinical.

First, there's the question of the strain. Most practitioners recommend a softer mushroom like Golden Teacher in the family *Psilocybe cubensis*. At medium to higher doses, average humans should take roughly three to five grams, depending on body weight and past sensitivity. If you have no past experiences, you're going to want to take it easy. If you're not feeling anything immediately, probably one of the worst things to do is take another handful outright. Many suggest drinking orange juice or other citrus including so-called lemon tek. Lemon tek requires a bit of planning as you soak ground mushrooms in a glass of lemon juice before drinking down the mix. The belief is that this technique improves absorption and reduces the bitter taste of the mushrooms.

Still not feeling anything? Give it time and understand that some trips aren't meant to be.

Folks commonly report an onset within the first hour. Early sensations can include yawning, light queasiness, shifts in temperature, and an elastic sense of time. You can increase the chances of a trip by stimulating the vagus nerve through low chanting or humming, although you might feel silly. Over the next hour the intensity rises. Music and touch can feel vivid, and many people prefer to lie down with eyes covered to lean into the experience. The peak often arrives around hours two to three, with strong changes in perception and thought. This can be blissful, challenging, or both. Your sense of self may loosen, which can feel expansive or unsettling. After that, most people move into a plateau and gradual descent, with softer visuals and a more reflective mood, followed by a calm afterglow that makes rest easy.

If you're a first-timer, please don't eat a handful and go wandering some botanical garden or to a Pink Floyd laser light show. Your goal is to create a container, a place where you can feel safe. In mushroom practitioner speak, this is a safe place that you will not leave during the experience. Facilitators will explain that they will hold the container for a set number of hours and will ask you not to leave during that time. If you come off your trip before the container, you'll be asked to wait quietly while everyone else is working through their dosages. If you're doing it alone, then prepare your own container by having a set time you expect to stop, say six hours after your dose, and planning to do nothing—no food orders, no video games, no livestock tending—for that entire period.

Put your phone away. Turn it off and hide it. Turn off all other devices in the house that can make noise or annoy you. Street noise or natural noise is fine, but you don't want an alarm clock to start blaring. Turn on a six-hour playlist. You can find plenty of them online, including ones designed specifically for tripping. If you're using Spotify or YouTube, maybe pay for a subscription so you don't get commercials in the middle of the trip. Nothing sounds weirder than a McDonald's jingle while you're flying through a neon field of digital emus.

You're also going to want to text people during your trip. Don't do it. Put a little notebook next to your bed if you must but remember that anything you write won't make much sense. I remember one trip when a friend who was lying next to me kept asking me, "Should I write this down?"

"If you want," I said. I was already coming down so I could speak clearly.

"But should I?"

"You need to do what's in your heart," I said, seeing her aura float above her like a purple candle.

She did and it didn't make any sense when she read it later.

Most practitioners wouldn't recommend doing your first large dose alone but it's doable with the right mindset. If you're doing mushrooms alone, prepare yourself for a long trip as described above and do not leave your container. Again, I reiterate: The throes of a mushroom trip are not the ideal time to do a little shopping or pick up some dry cleaning. I recall one experience in college where I took a heroic dose, probably four grams. I wasn't feeling anything and began wandering my neighborhood. I ran into some friends who were planning a party that day and they reminded me that I was supposed to go with them. I smiled vacantly and nearly wandered off until they asked if I was high. I was.

We then went to Eat'n'Park in Pittsburgh, a local fast-casual eatery. I was a vegetarian, so I ate only French fries. The fries had a crisp outer layer, a soft interior, and just enough salt. This was, I assure you, the first and last time an Eat'n'Park meal was truly resplendent.

Worried about what to do instead? Turn on some jazz or EDM. I love music on mushrooms. I've noticed that when listening to jazz or electronic dance music, I'm able to listen between the notes, noticing new sounds that aren't normally available to us. You'll hear fingers on guitar strings, a singer taking a quick breath, a series of notes that sound otherworldly. Techno, of all things, sounds less like a cacophony of sounds and more like an ordered selection of notes woven into luminous fabric. I highly recommend a nice mix of tunes during your experience.

Prepare your space by clearing a path to the bathroom. If you are doing a first higher dose, a trusted, sober sitter is wise. Their job is simple. They must keep you physically safe and let the experience unfold. All they have to do is read a book while you wiggle around on your yoga mat.

Eat light earlier in the day, then give your stomach a few hours before you start. Heavy, fatty meals can make nausea worse, and a completely empty stomach can heighten anxiety. Ginger tea or capsules may settle things.

Psychedelic mushrooms are food and they are digested just like non-magic mushrooms. You don't want anything interfering with the digestive process and you want to avoid visiting the bathroom often, especially since many find mushrooms to be emetic, which I learned the hard way on one trip. If you have the opportunity, cover the mirrors in your bathroom and avoid reflective surfaces. When we see ourselves under psychedelics, things can get weird.

Dress in soft, loose layers and have a pillow and blanket ready. It is common to feel chilly during the come-up and warm later, so layering helps you adjust without effort. Keep water nearby and sip occasionally. You do not need to force hydration. If you feel steady, gentle stretching or a slow walk to the bathroom is fine.

While you are in it, keep things simple. Begin lying down, breathe slowly, and notice what is happening rather than chasing it. If a wave of anxiety hits, extend your exhalations and remind yourself that you took something and that it will pass. Eyeshades or a scarf can open a vivid inner landscape. If that feels tight, soften the lights and rest your gaze on a calm point in the room. Avoid screens. They tend to fragment attention and can yank you into loops that are hard to exit.

Physical positioning can affect how a trip feels. If you are lying on your side in a fetal position, the trip will be more closed and intense. Try lying flat on your back with your hands facing the ceiling instead, allowing yourself to breathe and expand.

A few safety notes: Do not combine mushrooms with alcohol, stimulants, or other psychoactives. Keep sharp objects, car keys, and anything hazardous out of reach. Write down two reminders before you begin: *I took mushrooms. This will crest and pass.* If panic spikes, change one small thing. Sit up, take a sip of water, look out the window, or shift the music. If you or a sitter ever face a true medical issue, seek help. Go into an emergency room if you absolutely must. You can tell the doctors you took mushrooms. Clinicians care about safety first. Barring a high heart rate or fluctuating body temperatures, however, you are very unlikely to ever have a physical reaction to mushrooms themselves. The only dangers are how you react to the stresses and unique experience of tripping.

Here's how my trips usually go: When I take a standard dose I try to lie down immediately and cover my eyes. In most cases I'll listen to music and when I work in a group, I'll listen to the facilitator who might play DJ, musician, and psychotherapist throughout the night.

The first inkling that something is happening comes in the form of fascinating and colorful fractals that appear in my peripheral vision. Think about the patterns you make when you press on your eyeballs. Now imagine those same patterns as solid lines, objects, and figures. Sometimes you'll see faces, robots, and aliens. In short, your mind will conjure up things that are strange, exotic, and soothing.

As the trip progresses, the music and your hallucinations will blend together. You'll be able to see patterns in the music while they flash in front of your eyelids. You'll feel that your head has expanded to contain multitudes, and sometimes I sense that I'm in a larger room than I really am and that I'm alone. Many people report seeing and speaking to loved ones or spirits. I often heard my father's voice and saw my grandmother Sadie come back to me for a hug. You'll be crying sometimes, which is cathartic versus sad or scary. I just keep telling myself that everything is fine and that I'm safe, which 100 percent of the time, I am.

When you reach the peak experience, you might find yourself in a position of extreme vulnerability. I often feel like a child as images and thoughts whiz by. I'm always able to rationalize the experience, and at no point should you ever feel that you are unable to control yourself, but there is always the danger that you begin connecting what's in your head with reality. This makes it even more important to lie quietly and not move around too much.

Ego death on mushrooms is the felt loss of your ordinary "me," not literal death. At higher doses, many people report a phase where the familiar story of who they are, their body, and even their name loosens or falls away. It can start with fear and confusion, because the mind is stepping beyond its usual boundaries. With surrender, the experience often turns into a spacious clarity or unity, a sense of being more than the body and biography, followed by a gradual "coming back" with a new perspective on life. A practical way to say it: The rigid identification with "I" relaxes, sometimes collapses, then re-forms, and the afterglow can include less fear, more peace, and changed priorities.

I've experienced ego death once, something I'll describe in detail later in this book. I didn't enjoy it, but it helped me gain some vital clarity.

Therapists and researchers describe ego death as a death-rebirth process that can be frightening in the moment but transformative afterward. People may feel they are "going crazy" or disappearing into a void, then reach a point of acceptance, and from there move into relief, insight, and a softer relationship to control and certainty. Accounts include losing every personal reference, accepting "It's okay if I die," and returning with a lighter grasp on fears and attachments.

A crucial safety note from end-of-life and psychiatric work: Confusing the symbolic "death of ego" with biological death is a known risk in distressed states. The clinical remedy is education and support, because the psychospiritual death-rebirth, done safely, can reduce suicidal thinking. If you're taking mushrooms for a specific problem—alcoholism, PTSD, a terminal disease—then you should be working with a qualified practitioner. Please don't just grab some shrooms and hope for the best. You need real help from real people and I'm as far from a qualified practitioner as it gets: I'm a journalist.

If you are considering exploring this territory, a few guidelines help. Go in with clear intentions, not demands. Use a legal, safe container. Avoid psychedelics if you have a personal or family history of psychosis, untreated bipolar disorder, or if you are on medications that can interact with serotonin systems. Respect dose, since very high doses are far more likely to precipitate full ego dissolution and intense fear on the way through.

Finally, a word about bad trips. There is no such thing as a bad trip. Every trip is useful in some way. The key to any trip is curiosity. Many times folks experiencing a bad trip are actually experiencing the sense that they want a trip to stop and that the entire thing is too much to handle. There are two rules to remember: You are safe and the weird stuff is only happening in your own head and that nothing you see, hear, or feel can hurt you.

If you're having a bad trip, breathe. Remember that it will be over soon enough. Remember to be curious. Why are you feeling this way? Why are you afraid? Why are you reacting negatively? Answer those questions and you'll discover that maybe you're under stress or that you need a sense of control. The best advice? Lie back and relax and let the mushrooms do their job.

When you are coming down, aim for a gentle landing. Light food, a warm shower, and quiet time help the nervous system settle. Avoid big life decisions that night. Within the next day or two, write a few notes. What felt true. What surprised you. Name one small action you can bring back into ordinary life. That single step, more than peak fireworks, often determines whether the trip was useful.

Be kind to yourself. Perhaps you can even have someone ready to check in on you as needed, perhaps after six hours have elapsed. A good friend with some (washed) grapes and chocolate can be just the trick after a long trip.

A note on dose and variability is worth repeating. Three to five grams of dried *cubensis* is a significant experience for most people. Other species can be stronger per gram. Individual mushrooms in the same bag can differ meaningfully in potency. If precision matters, some people grind and mix a batch before weighing a dose to reduce variability. If that feels too technical, choose a conservative amount and lean on set and setting instead.

Finally, respect the red flags. Skip mushrooms if you feel pressured, if you cannot secure a safe, quiet space, or if you are trying to run from an acute crisis that needs support from people, not fungi. If distress lingers after the experience or you notice persistent changes in mood or perception, reach out to a qualified professional. The short version? Plan the container. Keep the inputs low. Trust that the experience rises and falls. Bring back one thing you can use.

Early on, I decided I wanted more context on the mushroom-taking experience so I spoke to practitioners and guides. One of those was Lizzie Snyder, a slim, intense young woman with long blonde hair who was framed by beautiful palm trees when I spoke to her. Snyder didn't set out to become a psychedelic practitioner. She was a neuroscience researcher prepping her PhD applications when a car accident derailed her life. Two blunt impacts, first from the side, then head-on, left her with a traumatic brain injury so severe she couldn't remember her own name.

"I went from applying to Yale and Princeton to not being able to spell my name or write the date," she said. "I couldn't even read numbers."

Doctors told her she'd never recover. They prescribed narcotics for the pain and suggested she accept a future of disability. But Lizzie didn't accept that. Instead, she built something new.

Her organization, Global Wellness, blends functional neurology, somatic therapy, and psychedelic medicine into one coherent approach for healing trauma and rebuilding lives. The model is designed for people like her, those who fall through the cracks of conventional care, or who burn out chasing stability that never arrives.

"There's a difference between trauma and the thing that caused it," Lizzie said. "The car crash wasn't the trauma. It's the residue, what lingers in the nervous system, the memory, the sleep, the body. That's what we work with."

She began her own recovery with hyperbaric oxygen therapy, acupuncture, and neurofeedback. But the breakthrough came when she introduced psychedelics into the mix, specifically ketamine, supported by somatic care and what she called "intentional frameworks." The psychedelics allowed her to reset. The structure kept her anchored.

In the sessions that followed, Lizzie didn't just recover. She restructured her life. From the fragments of her own injury came a new philosophy: Care must be multimodal, reciprocal, and, above all, accessible. If a client can pay, they subsidize someone who can't. If someone has resources, they share them. If someone's healing, they bring others with them.

And always, she said, the body leads.

"Breathwork. Coughing. Simple vagus nerve activation. These are tools anyone can use, every day," she told me. "Trauma sits in the nervous system. You don't need a spiritual awakening to address it. You need consistency and a map back to your body."

The work is especially relevant to those who grind themselves into illness, entrepreneurs, caregivers, people who are always one project or one disaster away from collapse. Lizzie didn't reject Western medicine. She used it. She simply went further, looking where the system didn't.

"The traditional model ran out of ideas," she said. "So, I looked elsewhere. And what I found worked."

Lizzie's approach isn't about rejecting science. It's about updating it to include the nervous system, the body, and the possibility of psychedelics as accelerants, not panaceas.

Today, Global Wellness doesn't rely on ads or algorithms. It spreads through word of mouth. She calls it a "signal," one that travels through people helping people. That signal now includes breathwork playlists, integration circles, and shared language for reframing pain as a starting point for connection.

"To be human," Lizzie said, "is to have connection. That's the medicine we're trying to remember."

In her model, psychedelics don't sit at the center. They're one piece in a system built on reciprocity, awareness, and care. The mushrooms, like the breathwork, help her clients remember how to come back into themselves.

Her rules for that practice were plain. "We have a framework that we live by," she said. "We are authentic. We are vulnerable, by our own choice when we choose it's safe to do so. And we are accountable for our own behaviors." In a hard moment, it sounded like this: "Hey, I'm feeling overwhelmed right now. Can I take a minute?" Those simple lines, repeated in real time, were the fabric repairs that held a relationship together while the nervous system learned safety again.

Lizzie did not present psychedelics as a single fix. She used them to lower the noise so that the work of repair could happen. She built community structures to keep that repair going. "We write frameworks for retreats, safe frameworks, as well as integration with people individually, one on one, in groups, families," she said.

If you zoomed out, you saw a pattern that fits the wider mushroom story. The medicine helps people tell the truth. It loosens what is rigid, then hands the job back to daily life. It helps them find their breath, go to sleep, build accountability, and use kinder language. Lizzie said that the healing never stops.

"You don't go to yoga till your back stops hurting and then it's over," she said. "You change the way you live your life to be happier." For relationships, that looked like fewer defenses, clearer asks, and a nervous system that could finally stand down long enough to let love do its job.

Mushrooms are having their moment. Lizzie, and many of the other people in this book, are living this reality in ways that make us, to borrow from Radiohead, fitter, healthier, and more productive. Amazingly, the same molecule that turns our shroomie friends blue is the one now reshaping the mental health landscape, and I wanted to understand every aspect of it.

Stargazer

Mushrooms become only as potent as we grow them to be. Certain mushrooms have always produced psilocybin naturally but in quantities that, while effective, weren't quite what we're taking now. Humans and mushrooms live in symbiosis; we cultivate the ones we know work the best and they thank us for this cultivation by, as one Jamaican shaman I spoke to said, unlocking doors in our brains that are usually shut fast. Like cannabis, modern mushrooms are different than they were even a few decades ago thanks to human intervention.

To test this theory, the next batch I grew was called Stargazer. I have a photo of the mushrooms in one of their grow bags with stems and caps peeking out of the dirt like a crowded fairy village. One fully expanded mushroom has the whimsical shape and coloration of a floppy brown wizard hat à la Gandalf in *The Lord of the Rings*.

Among the many varieties of *Psilocybe cubensis*, the Stargazer mushroom holds a unique place in psychedelic history. Sometimes referred to as the Inca Stargazer, this strain is believed to have originated in the highlands of South America, particularly near the ancient Inca ruins of Machu Picchu in Peru. Unlike more common strains, Stargazer mushrooms are now considered rare, their historical significance adding to their mystique. The name "Stargazer" itself is said to come from the mushroom's cap, which tilts slightly upward, giving the impression that it is looking at the stars.

All that said, Stargazer sits at the strange intersection of folklore, marketing, and myco-meme. That tidy origin story—a discovery in the Andes near Machu Picchu—could be a bit of poetic fiction drummed up to sell a strain. Retail copy turns that into ceremony and antiquity, a "flesh of the gods" strain carried through time. It makes for great packaging. The paper trail is thin. Veteran growers tend to wave it off as a plain old *Psilocybe cubensis* wearing a romantic label, one more cube scooped from cow pasture and sold with a postcard of Peru. That said, it's a lovely thought that this strain has been with us for centuries.

All I know is that when I passed Stargazer out to friends, they had heavy and long trips, something that also happened with the other modern strains I grew, like Jedi Mind Fuck and Blue Meanies. When I ate one wet mushroom after clearing out my tub, I found myself feeling a familiar buzzing in my teeth and blue trails in my vision that indicated that if I ate even a little more, I'd be flying. Stargazers were strong.

What people see in Stargazer tubs is familiar cube behavior. Golden to caramel caps, sturdy white stems that bruise blue, decent colonization speed, and average to strong potency reports; nothing that consistently separates it from the broader cube crowd. Forum logs echo that, with growers reporting fast grain runs and ordinary shoebox performance. If there is a "look," it is just the classic cube look. In my experience, the Stargazers grew quickly and well and matured beautifully, even in the spore bag I nursed them in.

Unlike my previous grows, I left them entirely in an all-in-one bag where the mycelium grew through the grains at the bottom of the bag and then expanded into the dirt at the top, a shroomie parfait that created an enclosed set of mushrooms and multiple quick flushes.

Again, the most important story here is cultural. In my experience, the differences among named *cubensis* strains are interesting but hard to pin down in a reliable way. Some researchers would disagree, and they are doing the work to test that claim in the lab. Growers and a few community labs are running genetic and chemical assays on multiple "strains" to see what is signal and what is packaging. They sequence markers to check how closely related these lineages really are, then pair that with chromatography or mass spectrometry to measure the alkaloid mix. The usual suspects are psilocybin and psilocin. You also see smaller amounts of baeocystin, norbaeocystin, and sometimes norpsilocin. The ratios shift from grow to grow and for someone to say that one mushroom is more potent than another is difficult. Quite simply, your results may vary.

A little bit about the bouquet of chemicals you can find in a mushroom. When people talk about psilocybin mushrooms, they usually focus on psilocybin and psilocin, since those are the main active compounds responsible for the psychedelic effects. Psilocybin itself is converted in the body into psilocin, which activates serotonin 5-HT2A receptors in the brain and drives changes in perception. But many species of psychedelic mushrooms also contain smaller amounts of related compounds. These molecules are chemically very close to psilocybin and psilocin, differing by small changes in their structure, mainly the presence or absence of methyl groups.

Baeocystin is a close cousin of psilocybin. It is missing one small chemical group, which suggests it may act as a weaker or partial version of psilocybin in the body. Some researchers believe it could be converted into an active compound, possibly norpsilocin, though this pathway has not been clearly demonstrated in humans. There are no solid clinical studies isolating baeocystin on its own, so most of what is said about its effects comes from theory and anecdote. Some users report that mushrooms thought to contain higher levels of baeocystin feel slightly different, sometimes more mental or more emotionally charged, but that remains speculative.

Norbaeocystin appears to be even closer to tryptamine, one of the chemicals found in psychedelics. It may function primarily as a precursor in the mushroom's internal chemistry, or it could be the chemical the fungus uses to build psilocybin. There is almost no direct data on its psychoactive effects in humans, and it may have only weak activity at serotonin receptors, if any. Norpsilocin, on the other hand, is structurally very close to psilocin and has been shown in laboratory studies to bind strongly to the same serotonin receptors associated with psychedelic effects. However, it may be less stable in the body and could break down quickly, which might limit its overall impact during a mushroom experience.

In practical terms, most of the psychedelic effect of magic mushrooms is driven by psilocybin and its conversion to psilocin. The other compounds are present in much smaller amounts and remain poorly studied. They may subtly shape the character of a given mushroom strain, or they may simply reflect steps in the fungus's chemical assembly line.

Some connoisseurs now talk about mushroom compounds the way cannabis enthusiasts talk about terpenes. In cannabis, limonene is linked to a bright citrus note and an uplifted mood, while myrcene carries an earthy, hoppy scent and is often associated with a more sedating effect. In a similar spirit, some mushroom growers and hobbyists pay attention to minor alkaloids like norbaeocystin or norpsilocin, selecting and breeding strains that may contain slightly different chemical profiles.

The science, however, is still out. Unlike cannabis, where terpene content can clearly shape aroma and sometimes influence the subjective feel of a strain, the minor tryptamines in psilocybin mushrooms appear in much smaller quantities. There is ongoing debate about whether they meaningfully change the character of an experience beyond the effects of psilocybin and psilocin themselves. So, if someone tells you that one mushroom is materially different from another, you can chalk it up to a different experience, set, or setting.

As for flavor, chemistry does not rescue the palate. Whatever the alkaloid profiles, a mushroom generally tastes like a mushroom. They're earthy, damp, and faintly bitter and don't taste like lemons.

That said, we can say that terroir is important. A tub's chemistry is potentially important, although no one I talked to could give me a straight answer as to the extent. Substrate, temperature, light cycles, hydration, harvest timing, and drying all push the final profile around. Even flushes can differ. A flush is when the mushrooms grow to full size. In most cases, tubs can produce two healthy flushes before the substrate is exhausted. Two growers can start from the same syringe and end up with very different results simply because of the temperature or even the time they picked their shroomies. People often attribute these differences to the brand name on the bag but, again, what they are feeling may be a blend of chemistry, environment, and expectation.

Which brings us back to Stargazer. The name conjures a place and a promise of wild, thoughtful introspection. The measurable part, the chemistry and the genetics, is still being untangled and often looks interchangeable with other well grown cubes. The cultural part, the story we tell about what is in the bag, is powerful. It shapes what people expect to feel before they ever take a dose.

Thinking about this strain brought me to the many myths associated with mushroom culture. As we get closer to broader acceptance of our shroomie friends, what are some theories and, arguably, crackpot ideas, that gave mushrooms a bad name?

First, there's the Stoned Ape theory, proposed by Terence McKenna in his 1992 book, *Food of the Gods*. It's not a scientific theory in the strict sense. There's no fossil record of mushroom use because, well, mushrooms are hard to fossilize, but it's a narrative that continues to shape how many people think about the evolutionary role of psychedelics.

McKenna's argument is straightforward: Early hominids living in Africa would have encountered psilocybin-containing mushrooms growing in dung-rich environments, especially those following grazing animals. These mushrooms, he suggested, had profound effects on the primate brain. At low doses, they may have sharpened vision, aiding in hunting. At higher doses, they triggered boundary dissolution, group bonding, and possibly the emergence of symbolic thinking. McKenna believed this shift in consciousness helped spark the development of language, religion, culture, and what we now call human self-awareness.

Mainstream science hasn't embraced the idea. There's no direct archaeological evidence of mushroom use in early hominid diets. Evolutionary biologists also tend to avoid explanations that hinge on a single thing. Still, the theory persists, not because it's proven, but because it's plausible in a poetic sense. We know that psilocybin changes perception and cognition. We know that humans have coevolved with plants and fungi in every part of the world. What McKenna did was take that basic fact and reframe human history through the lens of altered states.

Whether you find the theory compelling or not, it serves a purpose in this book. It opens the question: What role have mushrooms played not just in culture, but in cognition itself? Even if the Stoned Ape Theory isn't "true" in the evolutionary biology sense, it's pointing to something real, that human minds have always been shaped by the natural compounds they interact with. And maybe psilocybin, in some forgotten part of our ancestry, helped us remember how to think differently.

I asked Gordon Walker about the theory, just to get a read on what a real scientist had to say.

He wasn't a fan.

"There's a gene called FOXP2 that tracks with language development," he said. "You can follow it through hominid evolution. Language was a gradual process. Psychedelics didn't spark it overnight."

Still, I pressed him. Could psilocybin have shaped culture? Religion? Art?

"Maybe," he said. "But that's anthropology, and I'm not an anthropologist. What I will say is that psilocybin changes how we process information. It quiets the default mode network, the part of the brain responsible for ego and filtering the world. Without that filter, we see more. Not better, just more."

The default mode network (DMN) is a group of brain regions that become active when you're not focused on the outside world. It is what kicks in when your mind wanders, during rest, daydreaming, remembering the past, imagining the future, or thinking about yourself and others. You can think of it as the brain's background mode, always running when we're not engaged in a task.

This network includes areas in the medial prefrontal cortex, the posterior cingulate cortex, parts of the parietal lobe like the precuneus and angular gyrus, and the hippocampus, which is key to memory. These regions work together to maintain a sense of identity, narrative, and continuity. They help you reflect, simulate social situations, or replay old conversations in your head.

The DMN has become central to research on psychedelics. Studies show that compounds like psilocybin and LSD reduce activity in this network. When that happens, the usual boundaries that structure your sense of self, your inner monologue, your place in time, and your distinction from the outside world can weaken or dissolve.

Our brains live on shortcuts. They bundle reality into tidy packages so we can move fast. Rug. Bookshelf. Face. Street. Most of the time these summaries are helpful. They are built from habits, memories, and predictions about what should be there.

Psilocybin loosens those predictions because it binds to 5-HT2A receptors and shifts the balance between top-down models and bottom-up data. The brain trusts its shortcuts a little less and lets in rawer signal. Edges look sharper. Textures feel alive. Patterns repeat and morph. Music and color can blend. Time stretches or collapses. People describe it as seeing the world as if for the first time, not because new objects appear, but because the usual old label maker is turned down and sensation gets turned up. At one event I took part in, many first-time psychonauts reported seeing the world in 3D, as if it hadn't been in the first place. Sunsets looked glorious. Trees were covered in faces. The veil between fantasy and reality shredded and they experienced the world in ways that were glorious and disquieting.

Shroomies also change how the self is organized. The networks that keep our inner narrator tidy grow quieter. You can watch thoughts arrive instead of being carried away by them. The bookshelf is not just "bookshelf." It is wood grain, dust, titles, the space between the spines, and the feelings that come with all of it. Did you love books as a child? Did you spend an afternoon building a bookshelf for a lover? Did you experience an epiphany in an old library? All that can come back in strange ways. That extra input can be beautiful or overwhelming depending on dose, mood, and setting.

One popular admonition is to never look into a mirror on mushrooms. Why? One theory posits that our brains usually see our faces pink and full of life. On psilocybin, the brain relaxes its normal shortcuts and predictions. That includes the tidy template it uses for your face. In a bright bathroom with harsh light, the predictive model drops, and raw detail rushes in. Pores look like craters. Tiny veins stand out. Color shifts and shadows crawl. Pupils are wide. Muscle tone changes as your expression moves through micro-grimaces you never notice. The result can read as sick, old, alien, or not-me, which can spark a loop of anxiety.

Some folks even report seeing themselves as corpses.

These effects are not random nor are they particularly spiritual. They are chemical. It follows a simple idea. When the brain relaxes its certainty about what the world should be, it becomes more open to what the world could be. Perception gets richer. Meaning becomes more flexible. For some people that opens creative paths or new empathy. For others it can surface hard material that needs care and integration.

The current theory is that silencing the DMN allows for other brain regions to communicate more freely. That might explain the sensory blending, emotional intensity, and new insights people report during psychedelic experiences. It also suggests why psychedelics can sometimes break cycles of rigid thinking in conditions like depression or PTSD. If the DMN is the seat of the self, then psilocybin temporarily softens that seat, and in that space, something new can emerge.

Walker compared it to being a baby again. "Babies don't have a default mode network yet," he said. "Everything amazes them. A spinning mobile, a shadow on the wall. Psychedelics bring some of that back. They let us see leaves, not just a tree."

I asked if the revelations people have while tripping are real. He paused.

"One of the dangers of psychedelics is that they can feel more true than truth," he said. "You're wide open. If someone gives you a bad narrative while you're vulnerable, you can internalize it. That's how cults work."

What he was talking about was brain plasticity.

Mushrooms open the brain not with brute force, but with subtlety, like a key fitting into a long-ignored lock. Psilocybin temporarily softens the brain's default wiring and allows for new patterns of thought, sensation, and emotion. The technical term is neuroplasticity: the ability of the brain to rewire itself, to form new connections. Most of the time, especially in adulthood, that plasticity is dialed way down. We become creatures of habit, stuck in grooves carved by trauma, repetition, and the daily grind. Mushrooms disrupt that.

I noticed this in my early trips. I felt a certain kind of tenderness after, and I saw everything more clearly. When I came back from my first trip, I noticed that my city was brand-new. I noticed the concrete, the paint, the beauty and the decay of roof tiles that I could see in the 2:00 a.m. gloom. I saw smiles in every set of taillights, like each Honda Accord was winking at me. I was beaming, remembering music and hearing each song anew, at least for a few hours after the official comedown.

This rewiring leads to what some researchers call "entropy" in brain activity, a collapse of rigid patterns and a flourishing of new, exploratory ones. Under the influence, the default mode network, the system responsible for ego, identity, and the sense of self, goes quiet. That quiet creates space. And in that space, people often encounter forgotten memories, buried grief, unexpected joy, or what feels like cosmic insight. It's as if the doors of the mind swing open, just for a while.

But those doors don't stay open forever, and that's the point. The brain can't remain in a highly plastic state all the time, it would be chaos. We need stability to function. That's why these windows, of childhood, trauma, intense learning, or psychedelics, are rare and time-limited. They exist so that, occasionally, we can break out of the loop and do something different. They're not for escaping life, but for reengaging with it more fully.

One clinician I talked to said that psychedelics let patients open up in ways that were once impossible. Rather than hemming and hawing, offering excuses and explanations for behavior, they instead just dumped out language. They said what they meant instead of what they thought the psychologist wanted to hear.

In other words, psilocybin doesn't overwrite the brain, it loosens the grip of what's already there. And in that loosened state, with the right support, people can often do the hard work of healing, reframing, or even reinventing who they are.

In clinical therapy, psilocybin isn't just a chemical trip, it's a carefully structured experience designed to shake loose the mental ruts that many patients have been stuck in for years.

Clinical studies, especially those at Johns Hopkins,[1] NYU,[2] and Imperial College London,[3] have shown that a single high-dose session with psilocybin, conducted in a therapeutic setting, can lead to rapid and lasting improvements in conditions like treatment-resistant depression, PTSD, addiction, and, as we talked about before, end-of-life anxiety. What's striking is how fast it works, often within a day, and how long the effects last, sometimes for months.

During the trip, psilocybin disrupts that repetitive internal monologue that reinforces a person's depressive or anxious worldview. With the ego dialed down, people often describe feeling "connected to everything," or seeing their problems with unexpected clarity and compassion. There's room to grieve, forgive, reframe. Some describe it as ten years of therapy compressed into six hours. Others say it's the first time they've felt real hope.

But integration, the process of making sense of the experience afterward, is where the deeper change happens. That's when a therapist helps the patient map their visions, insights, and emotions back onto daily life. The brain, having entered a window of plasticity, is unusually open to new habits, behaviors, and beliefs in the days and weeks that follow. This is where therapy picks up: not to dissect the trip, but to build on it.

Most important, however, is that this model, one or two high-dose sessions, paired with weeks of preparation and integration, is fundamentally different from how we treat mental illness with daily pills. It's not about numbing symptoms. It's about facing them head-on and giving the brain a rare chance to rewire itself in the light of direct experience.

Back to wacky theories.

How about the one that posits Christianity was a mushroom cult?

That's John Allegro's thesis: Christianity, at its roots, isn't about a real man named Jesus, or even a new moral code. It's about a mushroom. Specifically, *Amanita muscaria*, that same red-and-white spotted hallucinogen that rich Siberian warlords ate and then pissed out for the serfs to drink.

Allegro was a lecturer in Semitic and Old Testament studies at the University of Manchester. Following his appointment to the international Dead Sea Scrolls team in 1953, he quickly became one of its most productive and controversial members. His training in Hebrew and Aramaic, plus a background in Oriental studies, suited him for the slow work of deciphering Qumran's fragments. His most famous early contribution was the Copper Scroll, a set of treasure listings hammered into thin copper sheets. Allegro produced the first full translation and publication in 1960, and for a time he was the public face of the Scrolls.

In 1956, Allegro also wrote a bestselling book, *The Dead Sea Scrolls*, that made him a popular figure in Biblical history and, more importantly, a lightning rod among more cautious colleagues. Over time, he was pushed to the margins of the project and ostracized by his peers.

After leaving the Dead Sea Scrolls team, Allegro began to argue that the early stories about Jesus are coded language for fertility rites and psychedelic mushroom worship practiced in secret cults of the ancient Near East.

The mushroom, for Allegro, was not just a pizza topping. It was divine. It grew without seed, sprang up after storms, and looked like a phallus emerging from a womb-like egg. Its effects—visions, awe, death and rebirth—matched the religious language of salvation and resurrection. Ancient languages, he suggests, are full of double meanings and wordplay that reveal a hidden mushroom cult: "Jesus" becomes a symbol, "cross" a pun on a mycological dismemberment. Even the Christian sacraments of anointing, communion, baptism, are interpreted as ritualized ingestion and veneration of the fungus.

To Allegro, the Bible is less a record of history and more a veil over ancient entheogenic rites. The mushroom wasn't just a sacrament; it was the god. Christianity, he writes, is a psychedelic mystery religion in disguise, one that eventually lost track of its origins and replaced sacred mycology with doctrine and dogma.[4]

This isn't a gentle theory. It takes apart not only Christian faith but the whole Western religious scaffold and suggests that what we now call "spiritual truth" may have once been rooted in the intense, unpredictable chemistry of a psychoactive fruiting body. Allegro saw the ancient world not as a place of moral awakening, but as a place where words, sex, and fungus collided in ecstatic experience, and we've been mistranslating it ever since.

When John Marco Allegro published *The Sacred Mushroom and the Cross* in 1970, he detonated a cultural grenade. Allegro made money, but he lost standing. Reviews called the work a "farrago of nonsense," scholars showed his Sumerian roots were largely inventions, and pointed out that fly agaric and its host trees do not even occur in the biblical Middle East. Fourteen British academics, including his former mentor, publicly condemned the book. One critic said it might be the "single most ludicrous" work of biblical scholarship ever published. Others called it careless, speculative, even dishonest, accusing Allegro of misreading ancient texts or citing sources that didn't exist in the form he claimed.

Allegro soon stepped down from his post at Manchester. The scandal outlived the scholarship, and the man who once popularized the Scrolls ended with his reputation in tatters.

The media didn't hold back either. *Time* ran a piece mockingly titled "Jesus as Mushroom." They painted Allegro as a fringe figure chasing psychedelic fantasies, a philologist gone rogue. His publisher eventually distanced itself. His academic career was over. Once a respected translator of the Dead Sea Scrolls, Allegro found himself exiled from the scholarly world, written off as a maverick who'd traded rigor for shock value.

And yet.

Like a mushroom spore waiting for the right conditions, his ideas didn't die. They lingered. In underground circles, among psychonauts and rogue historians, Allegro's theory kept popping up. Carl Ruck cited him. So did Terence McKenna. Today, you'll still find *The Sacred Mushroom and the Cross* on the bookshelves of curious mycophiles, psychonauts, and conspiracy-minded seekers. Why Dan Brown, he of the *Da Vinci Code*, hasn't written a thriller about it yet is a mystery although his latest, *Secret of Secrets*, touches on the idea of altered states.

Most serious scholars still reject it but the question he dared to ask, what if religion came from inside us instead of outside, was fascinating.

Allegro died on February 17, 1988, his sixty-fifth birthday, at his home in Sandbach, Cheshire. The controversy never really died with him, and the book still cycles through revivals and rebuttals.

The final weird mushroom story is the age-old tale of mushroom users harming themselves and others. As we said before, psychedelics used to be called psychotomimetics. The idea was that by taking things like LSD, researchers could re-create the experience of schizophrenia, dementia, and depression. That most of these ailments were nothing like a mushroom trip didn't matter: Any kind of alternative brain function was seen as negative.

A quick search for "mushrooms" and "suicide" brings up a few harrowing tales of psychonauts who seemingly took too much. In May, 2017, a student from Singapore took psilocybin in a Bali hotel and jumped five floors to his death.[5] A year earlier, a twenty-three-year-old Merrill Lynch analyst named Alex Lagowitz fell twenty-six stories after eating mushrooms.[6]

"He was really high on mushrooms and jumped out the window," said a friend. Correlation, however, is not causation.

Stories like these surface every few months, then get folded into the usual narrative about dangerous drugs. A *New York Post* source even offered the old line that mushrooms can make you believe you can fly like Superman.

Psilocybin can absolutely distort perception. People have been hurt, even killed, while under its influence. That is true. It is also true that, in large population surveys, mushrooms look comparatively safe as recreational drugs. In the 2017 Global Drug Survey, about ten thousand people reported using mushrooms in 2016 and roughly 0.2 percent sought emergency care. That rate is several times lower than LSD, MDMA, cocaine, or alcohol, and lower than cannabis. Both things can be true at once.[7]

So, are mushrooms going to send you into traffic, or are they safer than a night at the bar? The answer depends on who you are, how much you take, where you are, and whether anyone is looking out for you.

Most researchers draw a clear line around psychotic spectrum risk. A personal or family history of schizophrenia or bipolar disorder raises the chance of a serious adverse reaction. There is no good evidence that psilocybin causes schizophrenia, but if you are already vulnerable, the experience can unmask or worsen symptoms. That is enough reason to be cautious.

Darrick May at Johns Hopkins, who works on psilocybin research and harm reduction, told *Vice* that the field has moved away from the psychosis-mimic idea, while keeping strict screening. He also noted that bad outcomes in the wild often have two features: an unsafe environment and unknown histories. At a festival, no one knows your family's mental health background. If you combine a high dose with heat, dehydration, stimulants, or a balcony, you have stacked the deck against yourself.

Bob Jesse, a coauthor on a large study of difficult psilocybin experiences, found something similar. Nearly two thousand people described their hardest trips in a rigorous online survey. Even at that scale, the data could not cleanly predict who would have a rough time from demographics or self-reported history alone. Serious incidents are rare, which makes them hard to model. The field's working rule remains simple. If you have a personal history of schizophrenia or bipolar disorder, do not take psychedelics.

In clinical studies, well-screened volunteers take psilocybin in a quiet, supportive room with trained monitors. They prepare for the day, then integrate afterward. Under those conditions, severe events are uncommon. In the real world, people dose in hotel rooms, busy streets, rooftops, and clubs. Most of the worst stories are not about toxicity. They are about context, co-use with other substances, and ignoring basic safety.

None of this is a defense of careless use. It is a reminder to separate moral panic from useful caution. Mushrooms are not a party drug, even though many treat them like they are. The bottom line? Treat them with respect.

Penis Envy

Mushroom names are frustrating. On one hand, they can be perfectly precise, as if some enlightened psychonaut looked hard and called the thing exactly what it was. Some are tied to geography, the places they came from: Acadian Coast, Malabar. Others, like Golden Teacher, nod to the trickster gods tucked inside the hyphae. Then there are the names that feel like they were chosen by someone with less poetry in the tank. The particular shaman who named Penis Envy picked it for one obvious reason.

As it grows, it looks like a wiener.

Penis Envy is the one people whisper about in retreat circles and on message boards. It is the "strong" one, the strain that will knock you on your butt. It does not look like the others. The stems are thick and stubby, the caps are round and often never fully open. It looks more like a glitch in the species than a clean, textbook mushroom strain. It tends to drop far fewer spores than normal cubes, which makes it harder to propagate and adds to its legend. Growers depend on tissue cloning and liquid culture, passing the line from hand to hand. Taxonomically, it sits inside *Psilocybe cubensis* as a cultivated variety, but in practice its growth habits and body shape set it apart from the rest of the family.

The origin story is one of the most tangled and retold in psychedelic lore. For years, the go-to version was a 2009 *Vice* piece[1] by Hamilton Morris, which traced the mushroom to Terence McKenna's wanderings in the Amazon. In 2021, Morris said he had been misled by the infamous mycophile John "Mushroom John" Allen and by half-true rumors on early forums. The real story, as later pieced together, is stranger and messier.

The trail still began in the Colombian Amazon. In 1971, Terence and Dennis McKenna stumbled on a wild patch of *cubensis* while chasing the visionary *oo-koo-hé*, a brew containing N,N-dimethyltryptamine, or DMT. This compound, closely related to psilocin, was found in various plants and had been discovered in a legendary preparation used by local groups to see spirits. The brothers also searched for, according to Morris, "a mysterious blue ectoplasm that gushed from the mouth, anus, and genitals of shamans in the midst of drug-induced trance states," which they decidedly did not find. Instead, they brought several spore prints and mushroom samples back to Colorado, including one weird and girthy sample that evaded spore printing. That sample, passed along through the underground, eventually reached Steven Pollock, a physician who quit medicine to go deep into the mushroom world. Pollock was often credited with isolating a mutant lineage that grew thick stems, kept caps tight, and hit unusually hard. Because it looked like a comically erect member, he called it Penis Envy.

Pollock was the author of a rare book called *Magic Mushroom Cultivation* and laid out methods that growers still follow, including using brown rice to coax out fruit with high psilocybin content. He isolated a strain that produced unusually large sclerotia. These are dense fungal knots that could be stored, shipped, and consumed where fresh mushrooms were illegal.

Pollock was also a visionary. He wanted to set up the first legal lab for medical mushroom research and thought two million dollars would make it real. With a partner, he created a company called Hidden Creek in 1979 and began selling *Psilocybe tampanensis sclerotia* by mail through ads in *High Times*. Within a year, Hidden Creek was the largest magic mushroom vendor in the world. At the same time, he planted cannabis to bankroll his research and traveled through Mexico and the Amazon, returning with three new species, *Psilocybe armandii*, *Psilocybe wassoniorum*, and *Psilocybe schultesii*.

The pressure built. He had a medical degree, and Pollock's prolific prescription writing drew state scrutiny. Instead of stopping, he allegedly bought a pharmacy to supply his customers directly. By early 1981, his operation allegedly included nearly two thousand jars of psychoactive mushrooms growing in a San Antonio greenhouse. Then it ended. On the evening of January 31, 1981, Pollock stayed late at his office. He spoke to his girlfriend, told her he had a patient coming, then cut short a call from Paul Stamets. Hours later, she found him dead, shot in the head, the office ransacked. Police dumped and burned his entire grow.

Investigators later suspected three men, patients and a meth dealer among them, but the case was never prosecuted. The district attorney's role was disputed, records were destroyed, and Pollock's murder remains unsolved. Some even believed that Pollock died with a sample of Penis Envy clutched in his hand, a strange addition to a stranger tale.

For years, the story stopped there. Then a surviving spore print labeled simply "penis" surfaced. Hamilton Morris followed it not to Pollock but to Rich Gee, a Washington-based cultivator and genetics tinkerer who had quietly kept the strain alive. Gee, born Richard Gutierrez, published two obscure cultivation books, including *Cubensis Aquarium Gardening* in 1995. That small-run manual reportedly showed the first published photo of the then-unnamed Penis Envy. In an interview, Gee said the spores traced back to McKenna's Amazon collections, although he never met McKenna.[2] He received them through his coauthor, Jules Stevens, a Seattle hairdresser connected to one of McKenna's contacts. Gee refined the line through cloning and careful selection, preserving the mutation that became Penis Envy.

Put simply, McKenna brought spores and samples home. Pollock popularized a mutant line and gave it a randy name. Pollock died before it spread widely. Gee kept it alive in the shadows and left just enough breadcrumbs for someone to reconstruct the path. Out of accident, obsession, and hearsay, PE became one of the most potent and mythologized mushrooms on earth.

Penis Envy grew in popularity. In the 1980s and 1990s, when samples filtered through the underground, people learned fast that a "modest" dose could feel immodest. Reports and sporadic lab assays had long put it on the high end of *cubensis* potency, sometimes two to three times the alkaloid content of garden-variety cubes. The stories spread in rave scenes and on early forums. Someone ate two grams thinking they were cruising. They were not cruising and instead experienced full ego death.

Even years later, facilitators told PE first-timers to start small. People described PE as heavy in the body and unforgiving in the head. Visuals stacked up. The interior space felt vast. The lessons could be sharp. Compared to Golden Teacher's warmth or Liberty Cap's playfulness, this one had a reputation for grabbing you by the collar. It was not a mushroom that taught gently.

Over time, offshoots appeared, each with its own quirks. Albino PE, with its ghost-white caps, was a popular contender, and Uncut PE, with even tighter veils, began to enter the market. PE6 and other crosses tried to blend potency with more reliable spore production. None had knocked the original off its pedestal. What started as a mutation turned into a symbol of how unpredictable fungi could be. It was also a reminder that human hands shaped fungal futures. We named them, cloned them, traded them, and, sometimes without meaning to, helped them evolve.

A final practical note for readers who did not live on message boards. "Strain" names for *cubensis* were folk taxonomy. They were useful labels inside the community, not formal botanical categories. Potency varied wildly from grow to grow. What one person called "PE" might have been a faithful clone of an old line or a recent cross that resembled it. The stories we told about these mushrooms traveled faster and farther than the mushrooms themselves. That was part of the magic and part of the problem.

I wanted to give PE a go, so I ordered my next syringe and prepped my grow.

To grow my PE, I turned to a newer and much simpler tool for cultivation, the spawn bag. At first glance it was just a plastic pouch full of rye or another sterilized grain. In practice it was a small ecosystem. The plastic was heat resistant. A filter patch let fresh air exchange while keeping microbes out. Once sealed after sterilization, the bag became a ready-made incubator where mycelium could run through the grain without being smothered.

What was most important about the spawn bag was that it was completely self-enclosed, much like a hunk of mycelium would be when trapped in the middle of a compost pile. Furthermore, the environment was clean. Everything from the rye berries inside to the bag itself was sterilized and microbes were kept to an absolute minimum.

Spawn bags mattered because they lowered the barrier to entry for growers. You could even buy spawn bags with built-in substrate, allowing you to grow mycelium in the bottom portion of the bag and, when the mycelium was ready, break the whole mess up and start growing the mushrooms in a layer of prepared substrate. These two-in-one bags were popular with culinary mushroom growers who expanded the mycelium and then "sent" or fruited their bags, essentially forcing them to begin producing shroomies, by ripping off the top and letting oxygen and light hit the substrate.

With PF Tek, growers cooked jars of brown rice flour and vermiculite, sterilized them in pressure cookers, and worried about contamination at every step. Jars worked, but a bad seal or a rushed process could ruin weeks of effort, and pressure cookers sometimes failed with messy, scary results. Most growers didn't want to put a bunch of glass under pressure, no matter how easy it seemed. With a bag, most of that risk and fiddly work moved upstream. After inoculation with spores or liquid culture, the only real ingredient left was patience.

Bags also changed the scale of growing. A single bag held far more grain than a jar, so you got more mycelium to expand into bulk substrates. That could mean bigger harvests and less waiting between flushes. For commercial operations, bags became standard because they were stackable, inexpensive, and easy to move from incubation to production without juggling racks of glass.

Matthew McInnis of North Spore watched the spawn bag craze roll in like a tide and knew exactly how to surf it. McInnis and team leaned in, turning presterilized grain and bulk into a consumer product. Branded sterile substrates and filter-patch spawn bags became the on-ramp. Behind the scenes they invested in automation to hydrate, mix, fill, seal, and cook at scale, so the bag that arrived on a Tuesday in Tulsa matched the one that shipped on Friday from Maine. The value proposition was simple. Bags were cheap, easy, and fast, and they worked.

That combination of access and restraint became the brand. North Spore made it easy for first-timers to get a clean run with a bag and a simple kit, while keeping their public stance focused on mushrooms in general. They even put time into replicating legends, like the old tryptamine-fortification study, and told people what the data showed. McInnis did not need spawn bags to define the company. He used the wave to grow a durable business that still worked after the froth blew off. Spawn bags turned a fussy and weird mushroom-growing system into something that anyone could do.

There was a symbolic shift in there, too. The spawn bag marked the move from kitchen-counter tinkering to something closer to agriculture. It industrialized what used to be an intimate ritual of boiling jars and peeking into cupboards in the dark. Some saw that as progress. Others saw it as a step away from the romance of cultivation. Either way, spawn bags had become part of the story, an invention that opened the door for people who never imagined themselves hovering over a pressure cooker or watching a dozen mason jars.

Once the culture touched down, the first threads slipped out like feelers. Hyphae tested the neighborhood, tasted the starch, and started releasing enzymes that turned hard grain into something sippable. A day later, the white showed up at the edges, soft and tentative. Then it started moving with intent. Every kernel that got wrapped became both food and scaffold. The network kept branching and returning to itself, fusing and cross-stitching until the bag looked like it was filling with frost.

The bag breathed all the while. Oxygen trickled in through the filter. Carbon dioxide drifted out. That exchange set the mood. High CO_2 kept the organism in builder mode. Low CO_2 and a whiff of the outside world said fruiting was near. Until then it was pure construction, a civil engineer with a sweet tooth.

Once a spawn bag was fully colonized, the shroomies were ready to be sent. The bag took on a marbled look, like a white mortadella, with grains embedded in a solid loaf of mycelium and the occasional amber spot. Anyone who stuck with this long enough would notice it, golden or tea-colored liquid pooling in a corner of a jar or bag or weeping from a tired substrate. Growers called it mycelium piss because the nickname fit what it looked like, a strange fungal urine seeping from the white network.

What was happening was less crude and more interesting. The liquid was a mix of metabolites, the chemicals a fungus exuded when it was stressed or defending its turf. When mycelium sensed bacteria or mold, or when conditions were just a little off, it secreted compounds that helped it break down competitors or cope with the environment. It was a simple immune response. The gold color came from those concentrated metabolites, not unlike how our bodies changed fluids during an infection.

A little metabolite was normal and usually harmless. It often showed up when a colony had sat too long or the substrate ran a bit wet. If the mycelium was otherwise bright and vigorous, it would keep marching. A lot of liquid, or a foul odor riding along with it, was a warning that contamination might have taken hold. Experienced cultivators read metabolites like weather signs, sometimes as a gentle nudge to move things along, sometimes as a signal that a project was better retired. Either way, it was a reminder that fungi were alive and responsive. They were not passive lumps waiting to fruit. They were busy organisms making chemical decisions about survival.

A spawn bag might not have looked like much for a long time, but inside it was all weather, traffic, and appetite. The filter patch was the lung. The grains were the city blocks. The whole thing was a tiny planet with one ambition: to turn food into living fabric.

The core of a busy bag ran warmer than the room, so condensation beaded up, rolled, disappeared, returned. Shroomies loved that heat because it felt like the core of whatever rotting thing they had chosen to live in. Most grew in dung, so a dense, very hot mass of organic matter was home, something they could slowly eat and expand into.

If you watched the spawn bag long enough you started to notice patterns. The mycelium created its own network, one that started with a star of mycelium at the injection port, something that looked like an alien octopus clinging to the bag and rye berries, which then expanded into the heart of the bag. The mycelial network was not a mind in the way we thought of minds, but it did make decisions. It chose routes around tough hulls. It doubled back where the grain cracked just right. It walled off places it did not like. It edited its environment, nudging the pH, secreting compounds that kept competitors at arm's length although, logically, the bag should have been a sterile field. If something unwanted got a foothold, the bag started telling stories in color and smell. Sour-sweet and slick meant bacteria had thrown a party. Thread-thin gray that rushed across the surface was cobweb. Sudden green was the old enemy Trich that won on speed. When everything was right, it smelled like damp forest and fresh bread. Unfortunately, some of the bags I used were infected and even in the confines of their plastic prison my shroomies were overtaken and killed.

There was a tempo to the whole thing. At first you caught single hairs. Then you saw tufts. Then you saw sheets. The fast lanes, called rhizomorphs, pulled across bare patches and knitted them closed.

Under the white, the grains were changing. Starches were cleaved. Proteins were nibbled. Cell walls got softened. The bag was not only a container. It was a stomach and a workshop.

One of my favorite things was coming down daily and looking at my shroomies grow. They changed from hour to hour and sometimes a bag that was clear one day was completely white the next. It was always a surprise. I also learned that mushroom growing happened on the mushroom's timetable, not mine. Some bags lay dormant for weeks and then exploded, others didn't fruit at all. Barring a microscope and deep understanding of mycology, there was no way to tell what would happen.

On the other hand, some environments kept you waiting. For example, during the winter mycelium often grew slowly or not at all, resulting in empty bags. One batch I inoculated seemed to give the berries inside some kind of gray tinge which the folks at Midwest Grow Kits, another mycology supplier, said was mycelium. That batch never really took, probably because the environment wasn't consistently warm.

Once a bag was full you had to crack it, separating each mycelium-covered grain. These grains would then regrow and regroup, creating an even more robust ecosystem. When the little shroomie city got jostled, it behaved like a living fabric. If you tore it, it stitched itself. If you spread it, it claimed new blocks. Every new contact point was another breath, another budget of enzymes, another chance to turn brown into white. The whole bag was one organism that expanded its range.

What the organism wanted was simple. It wanted more edges. It wanted more places to grow. When it ran out, it started checking the sky. Light sneaked in through the plastic. Fresh air teased the patch. Moisture wicked and evaporated. Those were the cues that flipped switches. The white smoothed over into dense plates. Knots the size of grains of sand appeared where currents and textures intersected. The future bodies of mushrooms were written there in miniature, waiting for a cooler breeze and a better draft.

Most of the time, though, the bag was not a theater for fruit. It was a training ground. The point was vigor. A well-run bag made a confident network that could handle change.

There were small dramas that played out every day that never made it to Instagram. The way the white went translucent where it had eaten through and then returned denser than before. The way the bag hardened in your hands once the kernels were cross-linked by hyphae, as if someone had stuffed a mattress into a plastic sack.

Fungi did not hurry. They persisted. They approached problems from the side. They were generous where they were strong and guarded where they were thin. They left a little of themselves on every surface they touched, just in case. They did not need much to begin, but once they began, they wanted everything.

If you left a colonized bag alone long enough with the right whispers of air and light, it would try to finish the story it had started. It would push out primordia that pressed their faces to the filter patch, hunting for a draft. It would bruise blue where it was squeezed, a chemical sign that said the machinery inside was sensitive and alive. Most growers never saw that in a spawn bag because the next act usually happened elsewhere. But it was there, written in, ready.

Inside the bag the shroomie built itself one grain at a time, tied itself into a net, and waited for me to keep it going.

Over time the spawn bags finished out, and I was ready to move the PE where it needed to go. I doubled down on cleanliness, wiped the new tub with alcohol, plugged the breathing holes with fresh cotton, then opened the bags and poured in the bulk.

The bags gave off a scent like a barnyard full of portobellos. It was calming, the same deep-wood note I remembered from my father's mushroom hunts, when he came home with heavy, dark caps from the forest. What made it stranger was that this was coming from a fresh spawn bag. No pins. No fruit. Just a preview. A reminder that every stage of a mushroom's life is tied to the last, that the perfume starts in the engine room long before the blossoms arrive.

I crumbled the mycelium in the bag and cut it open. Then, while wearing blue surgical gloves, I mixed the substrate—the dirt—with the grains. At this point the mycelium was strong enough to shrug off a little competition, but I did not tempt fate. I tucked the rye berries out of sight under the dirt and kept mixing until it looked like white-chocolate-chip brownie batter.

From there the work was mostly weather simulation. When you grow mushrooms, you try to fool them into thinking they're going through a change of season, the kind that says time to fruit now. Mushrooms read humidity, temperature, and light like an alarm clock, so you give them gentle cues. Before any of that could matter, though, the mycelium had to claim the new territory and stitch it together again.

The process took about a week. The surface went from brown to patchwork to cloudbank, little continents of white marching toward each other until they touched and held. Here and there the texture shifted from fuzz to knots, and then to the tiniest pinheads, proof that the underground city had agreed on its next move.

If you watch closely in this phase, you can see the tub breathe. The walls fog and clear. Droplets form, slide, vanish, return. That's also the whole system sweating, a sign that the metabolism inside is still driving forward. And the smell, that calm, clean barnyard note, lingers as a promise that the fabric you cannot see is already being woven.

When the mushrooms entered the fruiting stage, I basically had to stay home. My PE moved fast once they committed, throwing up those unmistakable, penis-like clubs within a few days. The speed of it felt unnerving. One morning I saw nothing but a white quilt. By the end of the week there were thick spears where there had been only bumps.

Pins were the first sign that the mycelium had understood the new program. I gave it oxygen and a little light, lowered the CO_2 by wagging the lid of the box to let in air, and it started to build fruit. The pins looked like tiny models of the adults, small stems with darker caps that had not even thought about opening. They were adorable, and they were hungry. I misted daily to keep the surface from drying out so the mycelium had the water it needed to keep building. Mushrooms are mostly water. The network did not have veins, but it moved moisture through its hyphae and inflated tissue with pressure, which was why a tub could change so quickly between breakfast and dinner.

Day by day the shapes thickened and changed. The little nubs became sturdy stems and dense caps that felt surprisingly firm, more like packing foam than something fragile. Color shifted from the gloss of newborn white pins to the matte of mature caps. With PE, the caps often stayed stubby and tight, so I read other cues. The surface of the cap went from slick to dry. The stem took on that stretched look. A nick at the base bruised blue within seconds. All of it told me the body was moving water, sugars, and everything else it needed from the colonized grain into these new organs.

Fruiting turned out to be less about heroic intervention and more about steady attention. I kept the surface moist without pooling, kept fresh air moving without letting the whole environment dry out, and let evaporation do its work. My job was to watch the weather inside the box and to harvest at the moment when each fruit looked ready, which arrived sooner than I expected.

One thing that surprised me about growing mushrooms was how quickly the substrate shrank. Day by day I could see the block pull away from the sides of the tub. By the end of the first flush, it looked a size smaller, nearly a quarter down from where it started.

Most of that loss came from water. The fruits drank it and the rest evaporated as the mycelium warmed the block. Some of the mass left as carbon dioxide as the fungus digested the grain. The network also tightened the whole thing as it knitted itself denser, so the loaf compacted even as it dried.

The change had practical effects. As the block pulled back, a thin moat opened along the liner and encouraged side pins. These pins were a bit tortured. They had to push up and around the substrate and often smushed themselves against the plastic like a kid looking through a toy store window. This fruit was different than the mushrooms that grew free on top. The surface crusted in spots where I had not misted enough, and the interior felt lighter and tougher when I pressed a (gloved) finger to it.

Fully grown mushrooms usually send out spores soon after maturity. The gills on the underside carry those spores beneath a thin partial veil. When the mushroom gets large enough, the veil tears, a ring forms on the stem, and a fine dust settles across everything nearby. With PE, that moment often never really arrives. The caps stay tight and the spores are scarce. In my tub they barely dropped at all. I saw only a few faint flecks where a normal canopy would have painted the liner in cocoa brown.

The image of a whole flush ripening together felt both comical and a little obscene. Dozens of mushrooms tried to finish the same job in a plastic box the size of a few loaves of bread. It looked like a pollen storm trapped under a lid. I half wanted to carry the tub outside and let the shroomies cast their fate to the wind instead of dusting their neighbors.

Timing mattered in a new way that morning. The fruits felt dense and springy, like firm packing foam. A nick at the base blued fast. The veils on a few caps started to strain. I understood why growers talked so much about catching the moment. I took photos, breathed in that strange barnyard sweetness, and then did what the scene required before the tub turned into a spore party I would be cleaning up for days.

I harvested my PE and set them to dry with a kit I had bought from North Spore. The kit came with desiccant beads and a simple chamber, but it did not keep up with the volume of the haul. I switched plans. I ordered a food dehydrator on Amazon, loaded the trays, and ran it for about seven hours at 132 degrees Fahrenheit.

By the next day the change felt absolute. The mushrooms had gone from slick and heavy to cracker hard. Stems snapped cleanly. Caps felt light and rigid, like thin foam. The color deepened a shade and the smell concentrated into something close to cocoa and damp earth. The plump bodies I had picked now looked like wizened little wizard fingers, each one a small record of the water that had left.

After the first harvest I rehydrated the block and it swelled a little, but it never returned to its original size. Each cycle left it smaller, darker, and more spent, a record of how much food and water those hungry fruits had taken to build themselves. Most substrate blocks can handle two flushes. To get the second flush you have to dunk the entire substrate in water and let it seep, creating a lovely brown tea and a new set of happy pins.

That session marked the end of the run. The tub had done its work, and so had I. I looked at the trays and understood that I had finally seen a grow through from spore to harvest to dry fruits. It felt simple on the surface, but every step had asked for patience and attention.

So now I had a huge batch of very strong mushrooms, my first. What was I going to do with them?

I started with microdosing. My shroomies were supposed to help with my depression, and a full, eyes-closed journey felt like too much on a monthly or even quarterly basis. I just didn't have the time to lounge around on a yoga mat and listen to Leon Bridges for eight hours. A sub-perceptual dose felt more like a way to test the door than kick it in.

Microdosing is essentially the homeopathy of psychedelics but with a bit more credence to the art. Microdoses are basically tiny, almost imperceptible doses of psychedelic that you take on a regular basis, usually every two or three days, and that ostensibly improve your mood and functioning. As a dedicated microdoser, I can attest to this fact although, as we'll see, there is little real research to back up our claims. Microdosing did not arrive as a lightning bolt. It crept in from the margins, the way many ideas do, and only later picked up a name. In the 2010s writers and educators began calling it part of a "third wave" of psychedelics, a phase that favors measured, intentional use and integration into ordinary life rather than a stance against it. The aim was not to reenact the 1960s with heroic doses that left victims reeling for days. The aim was to bring small, structured doses into work, family, and health without blowing anything up.

Before we go deeper into microdosing, however, it bears bringing in a little real research. In a February 2026 article in *Neuropharmacology*,[3] a study led by Luisa Prochazkova attempted to test the microdosing hypothesis definitively. The news wasn't good.

"Microdosing psychedelics has been widely reported to enhance focus and problem-solving, sparking interest in its potential to treat attentional disorders such as ADHD," wrote the researchers. "However, existing studies largely rely on anecdotal evidence and lack adequate placebo control."

This study ran two trials, both randomized, double blind, and placebo controlled, using legal psilocybin truffles in a setting close to daily life. About 141 people followed a microdosing plan for weeks, not a single lab day. Some got active psychedelic truffles and some got placebo, and no one knew who got what until the end. The team tracked attention, memory, cognitive control, mood, well-being, and self-reported flexibility with standard tasks and surveys. After proper corrections, the results were plain: Microdosing did not beat placebo on the main measures. The researchers wrote:

> Contrary to expectations, microdosing did not significantly affect behavioral or subjective measures compared to placebo. While some initial effects were observed in social cognition, mood, and self-reported cognitive flexibility, these did not remain significant after correcting for multiple comparisons. Regardless of condition, participants predominantly reported their subjective experiences as positive, yet negative bodily feelings were enhanced in the active condition. Notably, participants remained effectively blinded throughout the trials.
>
> In conclusion, our findings do not support the idea that microdosing psilocybin reliably enhances cognitive or emotional functioning beyond placebo. Future research should explore individual differences in response to microdosing and

examine whether specific populations might benefit from targeted microdosing interventions.

So according to the experts, microdosing shouldn't work. But countless practitioners found that it did. Let's explore it, especially considering that most folks will want to try microdoses anyway before ingesting a full five grams.

The practice has roots in several older streams. Mid-twentieth-century researchers ran creativity and problem-solving studies with psychedelics, usually at moderate amounts. Those sessions brought engineers, architects, and scientists into supervised settings and produced early claims about focus, flexibility, and visualization. That body of work was not microdosing, but it set the table by linking psychedelics to everyday cognition.

For example, in 1966, Willis Harman and some colleagues published a study titled *Psychedelic Agents in Creative Problem-Solving: A Pilot Study*,[4] one of the clearest examples of proto-psychedelic research linking psychedelics to everyday cognition. The team recruited twenty-seven professionals, including engineers, architects, and scientists, and gave them moderate doses of LSD or mescaline in carefully structured, supervised sessions. Participants were asked to work on real problems from their fields rather than abstract puzzles, and they designed the environment to reduce distraction and encourage focus. The results suggested that psychedelics could enhance flexibility, visualization, and the "illumination" phase of problem-solving, with many subjects reporting fresh perspectives and producing solutions that outside judges later deemed useful. While limited in scale—only twenty-seven males took part—and shaped by the optimism of its era, the study remains a cornerstone showing how psychedelics might sharpen, rather than derail, certain forms of human creativity. In other words, small, Alice in Wonderland bites of mushroom could turn a humdrum math problem into a field of blossoming ideas.

After prohibition stalled formal research in the 1970s, the thread moved underground. By the 2000s, psychologist James Fadiman began collecting first-person reports at truly sub-perceptual levels. He and collaborators circulated a simple self-study protocol, gathered hundreds of accounts, and helped fix the vocabulary. When Fadiman published *The Psychedelic Explorer's Guide*[5] in 2011, "micro-dosing" entered the mainstream lexicon for many readers.

Fadiman spoke to several microdosers, including Stephen Gray, a "lifelong student, teacher, and researcher of spiritual paths, in particular Tibetan Buddhism and the peyote ceremonies of the Native American Church." Like many of the folks he talked to in his book, these microdosers were already on board with psychedelics and were more than willing to talk about their experiences. He spoke about taking small doses of mushrooms with friends while playing guitar, something that resonated with my Blues Dad mind. Gray said that he felt sharper and that his thoughts felt more expansive.

> One of the results of this sharpness was that my guitar playing became more focused and agile. I don't play guitar enough anymore to get through most songs flawlessly, but on those nights, my playing was definitely more on the mark. I also noticed that my ability to recollect lyrics was noticeably superior to my norm.
>
> In conjunction with the sharpness has been a softening of the heart, which helped me connect to the emotion of the songs. A lot of the songs I like to play have poetic lyrics that don't necessarily reveal clear and simple meanings. The songs of Bob Dylan and Leonard Cohen can be like that. . . . During these low-dose mushroom sessions, I've noticed that my mind instantaneously grokked meanings that had previously eluded me.[6]

Aside from a new appreciation of "Blowin' in the Wind," microdosing seemed to help people for no obvious clinical reason. A microdose is usually far too small to be perceptible in the psychedelic sense. You don't see visions; you don't hear voices. What people report instead is a slight shift, a sense that the wheels are turning more smoothly. For some, that small adjustment was enough to change the texture of daily life. Ayelet Waldman was one of them. She would later describe microdosing as one of the best things she had ever done.

Waldman has never been the kind of person who fit neatly into one role. She trained as a lawyer, worked as a federal public defender, and carried the weight of other people's mistakes and crimes into her own body. The job nearly broke her. When she walked away from the courtroom, she turned to writing, producing novels and essays that were sharp, funny, and often scandalous in their honesty. She married the novelist Michael Chabon, and together they built a life in Berkeley, raising four kids and juggling two demanding careers that fed each other as often as they clashed.

But underneath that picture of success, things were unraveling. Waldman slipped into a period of depression and self-doubt that bled into every corner of her life. Antidepressants dulled her but didn't heal her. Therapy gave her language but not relief. Lifestyle changes, exercise, meditation, diet, were no match for the cycles of premenstrual dysphoric disorder that battered her month after month. Her marriage grew fragile, her children tiptoed around her moods, and she could feel herself coming apart.

When she found James Fadiman's microdosing protocol, it felt less like a grand experiment than a desperate gamble. Every third day she placed a tiny drop of LSD under her tongue, one-tenth of a recreational dose, no bigger than a fingernail clipping. Not enough to hallucinate, not enough to lose control, just enough to see if something might shift. She described it as a quiet act of rebellion disguised as self-care.

Her book, *A Really Good Day*, is a diary of that period. Each entry records the slow return of stability. She wasn't talking to God. She wasn't seeing fractals. She wasn't wandering the desert looking for revelations. She was getting through the morning without snapping at her family. She was able to sit at the kitchen table and feel calm. She started writing again. That was the power of microdosing for her: not fireworks, not visions, just balance. A single good day in the middle of despair felt like salvation.

What makes Waldman's account resonate is how ordinary it is. She wasn't a kid at Burning Man. She wasn't a biohacker in Silicon Valley trying to squeeze a few more points of productivity out of her brain. She was a middle-aged mom in Berkeley, ordering an illegal drug from a friend of a friend and hoping it wouldn't blow up her life.[7] In between her diary entries she wove in the larger story: the discovery of LSD, the flood of research in the 1950s and 1960s, the collapse under Nixon's War on Drugs, and the slow reemergence of clinical studies at places like Johns Hopkins and NYU. But the heart of the book isn't history or policy. It's the reminder that sometimes one-tenth of a dose is enough to keep a life from falling apart.

The book blew the lid off microdosing in a way no scientific paper could. Waldman gave it a face, a voice, and a story people could recognize. As I expanded my own mushroom research, I learned that scores of people in my corner of the world were quietly experimenting the same way, tiny doses of LSD, little nibbles of mushrooms, not to get high but to feel steady. And it wasn't just happening in Brooklyn or Oakland. It was happening everywhere, across demographics and zip codes, whispered from one person to another, a small underground revolution moving by word of mouth.

The early mushroom work was small and a little scrappy, but it gave the movement shape. In 2018, a Dutch field study followed people at a mushroom microdosing meet-up and ran them through simple creativity tasks before and after their dose.[8] The changes were not dramatic, but they were measurable. Scores nudged up on both convergent problem-solving and divergent idea generation. It was a parking lot version of science—clipboards and truffles—but it put numbers behind what people had been saying for years.

Around the same time, researchers started asking microdosers to track themselves over weeks and months. Interview studies found the same pattern you heard from Waldman. Better mood. A little more energy. Work felt less jagged around the edges. But the effects were subtle, not guaranteed, and easily swamped by sleep, stress, and life.

When larger, more careful projects arrived, they showed how much expectation mattered. In a clever placebo-controlled "citizen science" design, volunteers took active capsules and placebos. Many reported feeling better either way. Expectancy was not the whole story, but it was a big part of it.

So, again, that first study we talked about found there was no real value to microdosing. But plenty of people have said the contrary.

As I began my own microdosing journey, I felt very little except a new gregariousness and a sense that things weren't terrible. That, alone, was more than I ever expected.

To understand the idea more clearly, I spoke with Cesar Marin, a former CNN sports producer who later became a calm, public voice on psychedelics. His story felt familiar, especially the part where he was laid off at the height of his career.

Whatever Marin was doing, it worked. When we spoke, he was beaming. The bright smile and easy manner were almost disarming. He was the kindest person I had spoken with in months, and the joy felt real. Coming from a pissed-off former journalist, that says a lot.

Marin spent twenty-five years producing live television. It was a grind that mixed urgency with routine.

"I was covering breaking news and was under a lot of stress. I dealt with a live shot that gets dropped. A guest that you had couldn't make it. . . . The story that you thought was your leading story, something else happens five minutes before you go to air and you must turn a whole show around."

The treadmill stopped when he was laid off. An entire life, an entire career, gone in an instant.

"I went from being a TV producer by trade to becoming an entrepreneur by necessity, by need," he said.

Psilocybin arrived just before the floor gave way.

"Right before I got laid off, plant medicine, psychedelics came into my life, and it completely changed things."

He did not come in seeking a cure. He was curious. He was also stuck in a cannabis habit that many told him was not a problem.

When he started with shroomies he tried microdosing. He started small and kept a schedule.

"It was through microdosing, the very small and intentional use of a small amount of psychedelics on a protocol, that things shifted," he said. "I was able to change my relationship with cannabis. I was able to say, *not right now. I'm at work. This isn't the moment.*"

The practice sharpened his view of what was coming. A slightly higher session pulled the future into focus. The media cuts kept coming.

"I became a number on a spreadsheet even though I had been there for decades." He stopped waiting for a rescue and began to act. He spoke about microdosing at work and people leaned in. Then he went to buy clothes that might spark honest talk and ran into clichés.

"Everything I came across was very trippy, very tie-dye." He saw the gap. "There's a need for an apparel brand that talks about psychedelics without it being weird, something that you can wear with a jacket, with a suit." He built Cultivating Wisdom and MicrodosingOver50, two websites dedicated to training and, in the case of Cultivating Wisdom, cool shirts. He wanted to start real conversations. He did.

He told me his favorite story. He stood in a supermarket wearing a Microdosing shirt, literally a bright shirt with the word "microdosing" slapped across it. He wore it to our talk and I ordered one immediately.

While he was wearing it, a woman walked up to him.

"You microdose?'" she asked.

"How can you tell? Because of my smile?" he replied.

Her reply was a rimshot.

"'No, because of your shirt, dumbass.'"

Then she opened up. Before microdosing "she would literally drink a bottle of wine every day," she said. Now, she was better.

"I microdose every third day. I'm more present for my husband. I'm more present for my kids. I'm more present at work." A shirt opened the door, and Marin was fascinated by the person who walked through.

Cesar is careful in how he speaks to people who ask for guidance.

"With psychedelics, I have conversations. I don't really make recommendations. I'll tell people what I did and how I used it and what it did for me." His advice to anyone facing a late-career pivot is simple: "Take inventory of who you are and what you're an expert at. What is your wisdom? What can you set as a buffet table of wisdom to cultivate a better future?" He used the skills he honed in the newsroom. He built courses. He aimed them at people who carry stigma or fear, people over fifty who want facts, not hype.

"We have honest, open, and objective conversations. This isn't about tripping balls. This is really about how do we become better humans," he said.

He is now building a next step for leaders who carry quiet stress. "We're creating something called The Summit Within with really small containers of five, six people. In my vision we're creating alternative boardrooms where you can do things that you can't do in a boardroom. You can't hug in a boardroom. You can't be vulnerable in a boardroom."

The aim is to shift focus from what he calls "F-you wealth" to "love you wealth," measured in the smiles you help create, not only in the zeros on a balance sheet.

None of this erased the hard days. He laughs at the myth that starting a company is easy. "It's not always smiles and rainbows. Those hard days are the days that really make you strong." What changed was the compass. Microdosing helped him quit daily cannabis, face a layoff with clear eyes, and swap a control room for rooms built for real talk. "It paved the way to reinventing my life," he said. "It changed my life for the better."

To gather the other side of the equation, I spoke to Tracey Tee, founder of MomsOnMushrooms and a stand-up comedian. Tee came to this after a collapse. COVID wiped out her live comedy business. A hysterectomy at forty-one pushed her into early menopause overnight. Wellbutrin helped. She did not want to stay on it forever. A friend took her camping and handed her mushrooms.

"They changed my life," she said. She taught herself all about shroomies and then built the thing she wished she had found, a place for mothers to learn together.

"We're an online educational platform and community that aims to bring mothers together around safe intentional use," she said about Moms on Mushrooms. Right now, the focus is microdosing psilocybin. She calls it a good foundation for people raised in a culture with no shared context for this work.

She rejects rigid protocols. "I don't really think that this medicine needs a protocol," she said. Her frame is simple. Start low, go slow, listen to your body, know your why. "This is like a co-created experience where you're required to do work," she said.

It is not Advil. It is not passive. You meet the medicine in the middle, she said.

Her first step for any woman is intention. Why now? What hurts?

"From mothers specifically, I hear, 'I just, I want to be more present with my kids,'" she said. Older women tell her they want to laugh again, or cry again, or stop feeling numb. Education comes next. She encourages microdosers to read, ask questions, and learn what they are taking and why.

"You've made it this far without shrooms," she said. "So, you can wait a few more weeks or a month while you read."

Tee is gregarious and has dark glasses and straight blonde hair. She looks like someone with a very arch view of the world and who, around the pandemic, spent time making people laugh. Now she pushes back on psychedelic fear with facts.

"We actually have no recorded known cause of death directly from psilocybin anywhere," she said. Risk comes from mixing substances and from unsafe choices, which is true for alcohol as well. She wants women to unlearn old stories and look at data with clear eyes.

On supply and laws, she stays careful. She will not coach anyone to buy. She points out that mushrooms are easy to grow and widely distributed in nature, then returns to education and community. Sharing the experience with other moms makes the learning easier and safer.

Tee's business is like Marin's. It's a community and it is large and growing. A private network called The Grow has about two thousand paying members. More than four thousand women have taken a course or joined a cohort in the last two and a half years. Some courses are self-paced. Others run in small groups for three months, with integration circles in between. The goal is to meet mothers where they are and to give them enough knowledge to make a real choice.

What do women report? Presence. Patience. Less reactivity. Less wine at night. More play with their kids. More creativity.

"I'm painting again, I'm writing again," are lines she hears often. She also sees promise in women's health, from PMS to perimenopause to postpartum strain. The science is still moving, but the signals for focus and mood are encouraging, especially when paired with daily practices like journaling or prayer or a quiet walk.

Her advice to women is steady. Know your why. Educate yourself. Go slow. Work in community. Do not expect a miracle. Expect work.

"Our job is really to educate mothers in the way that best suits them," she said. If that leads to a lifetime practice, good. If it leads to a clear no, that is fine too. The point is choice, informed and grounded.

Both Marin and Tee are the avatars for a new kind of psychedelic explorer. Instead of talking about digital elves and ego death, they are recommending small doses of very powerful and controlled medicines. Marin doesn't want us all tripping balls, as he said, he wants us to smile a little more and look and feel healthy.

What's unique about both Tee and Marin is that they have monetized their skills without being mercenary. Marin is selling T-shirts with a single word on them. Tee has a chat room and teaches classes. Neither of them are withholding sacred wisdom or pretending they are shamans bent on opening our third eye. They just want a guy like me to stop drinking so much and maybe not yell at his kids.

Today, microdosing sits at the crossroads of anecdote, commerce, and science. Community protocols and online diaries continue to shape expectations. Companies market premeasured mushrooms where they are legal and functional mushroom blends where they are not. Universities and hospitals are running controlled studies that will either validate parts of the story or narrow them. That is the history so far, still being written in real time.

There is a quiet shift underway among women in midlife and later, and it is not driven by pharma ads or weekend seminars. It is a slow, practical turn toward mushrooms. Not to check out. To show up. Mothers, grandmothers, caretakers, the backbone of families who carry calendars in their heads and everyone else's needs in their pockets. For them, psilocybin is starting to feel less fringe and more like a tool. Less about spectacle. More about stability.

It helps that the idea of small doses has a public record. Waldman's *A Really Good Day* did not try to sell anyone on cosmic revelation. She laid out a careful experiment with microdoses, tracked her mood, and described the results in plain language. Less reactivity. More room to choose her response. Better days stacked next to each other until the background hum of dread got quieter. For many women, that was the first time the conversation sounded like their lives.

Microdosing is not a magic trick. It is a rhythm. People describe it as a small nudge that lets them practice different habits with a little more ease. It is the difference between snapping at a kid and pausing long enough to hear the question. Between pouring a second glass of wine and realizing you do not want it tonight. Between scrolling and picking up a paintbrush, or a book, or a friend's call.

The changes people report are modest and human, and that is the point. Playing with the kids instead of supervising them. Music sounding like music again. A walk around the block that feels like a real break. A meeting where you say the thing you were afraid to say, and it lands. A pull back toward hobbies that were buried when life got loud. Not to monetize them. To feel a handhold again.

None of this is instant or easy. It asks for participation. It works best when it is paired with the unglamorous work of sleep, food, sunlight, movement, and boundaries. It works better with friends who will tell you the truth. It works best when you are honest about what is not working yet.

If there is a thesis here, it is simple: Microdosing mushrooms is not an escape hatch. It is a practice for returning. Older folks, at least folks in their forties and their fifties, seem to know what they want to return to. They want presence, patience, and a sense that time is theirs again. It will not happen by itself. But a small dose, a clear why, and a circle that holds you accountable can change the flavor of a day. Stack enough of those days, and you start to recognize yourself. That is not a revolution with fireworks. It is a quiet one, in kitchens and carpools and text threads. And, as Marin notes, it is enough.

Jedi Mind Fuck

The next shroomie in my collection was Jedi Mind Fuck.

Yes, you read that right. Jedi Mind Fuck, or JMF. It's one of the most notorious strains I ever grew, and it lived up to the name.

JMF is a cultivated, not wild, variety of *Psilocybe cubensis*, part of the long family tree of mushrooms that growers have been refining since the 1970s. "Modern" is a slippery word here. Unlike mushrooms with centuries of ritual use in Mexico or Siberia, JMF came out of the internet-fueled underground in the early 2000s. The name tells you everything you need to know. It promises strong visuals, an intense body load, and an experience that might leave you questioning reality. Cannabis breeders have Sour Diesel and Strawberry Cough. Mushroom growers went for a title that was less cute, more sci-fi. The intimation was that JMF would have you saying "These aren't the droids we're looking for" like some befuddled *Star Wars* Stormtrooper.

Like other *cubensis* strains, its roots trace back to wild genetics collected in Southeast Asia and Central America. Over time, these species spread through spore libraries, cloning projects, and message boards. As with Golden Teacher or Penis Envy, the exact point of origin is fuzzy. What matters is that it works, and that its reputation traveled faster than the mycelium itself.

Reports from forum users usually put JMF in the mid-to-high potency range. The trip is heavily visual with high color saturation, geometric patterns, and blue tracers across lights. People also mention a heavy body load that makes you want to lie down rather than wander around. Physically, the mushrooms are typical *cubensis*: caramel caps that flatten with age, white stems that bruise blue, and deep purple-brown spore prints. They have a bit more of that wild, fantasy-world shape with long stems and cute little caps that remind us of fairy forests.

Culturally, the rise of JMF is part of the bigger shift that happened in the 1990s and 2000s. The internet turned mushroom growing into a global community. Spore syringes, cultivation notes, and trip reports crossed borders in padded envelopes and on forums. Strains multiplied quickly, often with names meant to stand out in a crowded catalog. Traditional ethnomycology ties mushrooms to a place: Mexico, Siberia, the Amazon. JMF belongs to digital culture, born of message boards and spore swaps, a name dreamed up by growers trying to one-up each other.

And somehow, this name ended up in a government meeting. In Arizona, Dr. Sue Sisley and her team at the Scottsdale Research Institute fought for years to launch the first US FDA-cleared human trial using whole psilocybin mushrooms. [1] When the FDA finally funded their study in 2023, the team had to standardize a single strain. After fourteen grow cycles and forty lab tests, they chose their winner. When the state's Psilocybin Research Advisory Council asked what strain it was, Sisley deadpanned: "It's called Jedi Mind Fuck."[2] The room broke into laughter. The first state-funded mushroom trial in America would be run with a strain that sounded like it came out of a head shop on Tatooine.

The trial itself was careful and humane. Twenty-four participants received mushroom-dosed chocolates at varying strengths. The sessions included music playlists and even a therapy dog, an intentional nod to the mistakes of older psychedelic research. And importantly, Sisley pushed to study whole mushrooms, not just the isolated molecule. "When you extract one molecule out of the mushroom, you're taking out some of the intelligence, but you're leaving all the wisdom behind," she said.

My own encounter with JMF was interesting. At that point in my growing career, I had a ritual: Eat one mid-sized raw mushroom before drying the rest. It was my way of checking the batch. One afternoon, I picked a largish cap, maybe a gram and a half wet, and expected the usual light queasiness, maybe that strange sensation I always get where my teeth feel too big for my head. Instead, I had to lie down.

An aside about wet versus dry. Wet mushrooms are often less potent by weight than dry mushrooms. Mushrooms are mostly water, as we know, and the psilocybin is diffused throughout the fruit, meaning that a gram of fresh mushrooms is much less potent than a gram of dried. Furthermore, they taste different. Fresh caps can taste grassy and slippery while dried mushrooms taste more like morels, although some report them tasting muddy and dirty. Drying pulls off that water, concentrates what is there, and slows spoilage, though rough drying with heat or lots of air can oxidize some compounds and nudge the character of the experience. Dried mushrooms left in the light lose potency quickly and powdered mushrooms like those found in capsules can lose it even faster simply because there is more surface area for sunlight to oxidize the shrooms. Many growers and users say fresh can feel a little brighter and more somatic, dry a bit cleaner and more predictable, but the bigger practical difference is logistics. Wet mushrooms demand a fridge and quick use. You can tuck dry mushrooms into a jar with a desiccant and keep their potency far longer.

The visuals from JMF came fast. I got blue trails from lights and shifting textures across the room. Even though I took what most would call a microdose, it felt more like a mini trip on JMF. And because I had scheduled a podcast interview with a friend that day, I ended up on a call while still under its spell.

What happened surprised me. My friend talked about failure, about being an older creative in a world that no longer seemed to want him. And I listened, really listened, in a way I hadn't before. I poured my heart out too. The mushrooms had cracked me open just enough to let the words land.

The dose wore off quickly. I didn't become Luke Skywalker or Darth Vader. What happened was more interesting. A sliver of my heart opened while talking to a close friend. For all its bombastic name, that was the real power of Jedi Mind Fuck.

Thinking about JMF brought me to the idea of those Stormtroopers that Obi-Wan fooled on Tatooine. These things were powerful and were changing people's minds left and right, especially minds that were historically opposed to street drugs. That train brought me to another place where shroomies have become immensely helpful: in the world of PTSD sufferers who, despite often having a visceral reaction to street drugs, found precious relief after coming home from battle.

The stories are all the same: Something terrible happened while they served and they couldn't get out from under it. One woman I spoke to, Amy Charlesworth, a.k.a. QNAMY, made me cry.

Charlesworth is a striking woman. She has long dark red hair, regal cheekbones, and a manner so gentle and kind in the face of abject cruelty that the metamorphosis she experienced seemed impossible. But here she was, now a licensed psilocybin therapist in Oregon. Her story was horrific.

"I experienced sixteen years of abuse by the military," she said. "I was with the State of Oregon Army National Guard for the bulk of my career. They are, at least they were at the time, forty-ninth in the country for retention. So, the worst of the worst in all the United States for military service. The leadership is incredibly toxic. I dealt with some military sexual trauma situations.

"Just one example. I was over in Afghanistan and we had an internet service provider privately that two members of the S6 shop ran. They were in charge of the technology and communications department of the unit I was with. They were charging soldiers $100 a month for internet access into their rooms. And in order to connect to it, you had to give them the IP address off your laptop. And I didn't know how to do that. So, I dropped off my laptop. I was in my early twenties and they wiped my laptop of all my images and sold them for a hundred dollars per CD to all of the service members in my unit. These included naked images of myself. They were not held accountable. Being in Afghanistan, being in a war zone is so traumatic in itself. So yeah, a lot of different things. I did a lot of different roles in the military, human resources. I was a recruiter. I did some female engagement team stuff, jumping out of helicopters, air assault, and repel master. So, a lot of different things over sixteen years."

Charlesworth was so destroyed by her experience that she was ready to end her life. Before she tried mushrooms she began taking SSRIs, antidepressants designed to help mask the symptoms of depression.

"I had been on my first bout of SSRIs while actually in theater in Afghanistan. Even that initial experience with them was super inappropriate," she said. "The dosing was incorrect. I was drooling on the job due to the SSRIs on a cycle of sleep medications, taking crazy doses of Ambien, again inappropriately prescribed, and I became reliant on those. It messed with my circadian rhythm and my ability to manage my emotions and sleep and all of those things, it just became a toxic cycle.

"When I came home from Afghanistan, I suffered from extreme depression. I ended up getting a divorce. I had been sent overseas while my child was eighteen months old at the time. And so I'd been separated from him for well over a year and navigating back in the condition I was in mentally to being a wife and a mother just went south very, very quickly and the VA didn't have the appropriate type of support for that."

Charlesworth ran the full circuit inside the VA's mental health system. The plan was always the same: Try a new prescription, show up for talk therapy, hope something stuck. She stayed in that loop for close to a decade, fighting suicidal thoughts and waiting for a break that never came. She cycled through SNRIs and SSRIs, one after another. None of it moved the needle.

"And I got to the point where I was literally on the edge of killing myself. Like I cannot live like this. This can't be my death sentence," she said.

Like so many veterans I spoke to, she found salvation in someone who saw her pain.

"At an event that I was at, I had a conversation with somebody in the audience who had heard me onstage earlier say that I was suicidal. And they're like, 'Did you just publicly say you're suicidal?' And I said, yes. And they're like, that's not normal. And I'm like, I don't really know what normal is at this point, but this is my normal. And so they said, well, I know somebody that works with veterans and first responders, and they work with psilocybin and different psychedelics, and it saves their lives and the success rate is pretty profound, and I had not heard about these modalities before. This was the first exposure I'd had to them. And obviously being in the military, well not obviously, but being in the military, working with psychedelics or any kind of street drugs is so forbidden. You get drug tested frequently."

Two weeks later, thanks to a nonprofit that supported veterans and first responders, Amy was on a fully funded retreat. In one week, she worked with psilocybin, 5-MeO-DMT (Bufo), and MDMA, a.k.a. ecstasy. She walked out feeling like a different person. The weight she had carried for a decade, and pieces of her childhood hurt, finally slipped off. The psilocybin offered the long psychedelic trip and Bufo—toad venom—gave the quick-hit trips. Ecstasy evened things out, allowing her to work through the pain without going too deep down any dark holes.

"It seemed like my depression and my anxiety completely disappeared. My anger levels plummeted. My ability to deal and regulate my emotions vastly improved. And I've had friends and family members and peers kill themselves. And so I needed to lean into this all the way because my community needed this."

Amy's current mission is to get the medicines to as many people as possible, as quickly as possible. She talks about it on her podcast and is now a licensed facilitator, bringing what she learned to bear on others with the same problems.

What's important about this story is that it comfortingly but tragically repeats itself again and, in many cases, those suffering the trauma won't or can't get the help they need. That Amy and the countless other vets who used this medicine are still with us is a miracle, yet the stigma associated with mushrooms and other psychedelics is still strong.

What is really happening in these sessions? The science here is early for PTSD itself, but the signals are hard to ignore. In animals, psilocybin supports fear extinction and new growth in brain regions tied to learning. It's easy to feel this during a trip. Personally, I was able to examine anxiety I felt in a detached way. One special moment I remember involved a sense of panic that rose in my chest every time I thought of a certain moment in my life. The trauma kept coming back again until I lay in ceremony under about five grams of Golden Teacher. While I was under, I was able to instigate the panic and simply feel it.

"See?" I told myself. "That's all there is. It's not hurting you. It's not dangerous. Just feel it."

Of the dozen veterans I spoke to while writing this book, most of them experienced something similar. Basically, mushrooms let them look at their pain objectively and control it.

Studies outside PTSD show reduced amygdala reactivity during emotional processing. If your amygdala is always redlining, you avoid anything that feels like a threat, including memories. Turning the volume down may let a veteran stay with the hard material long enough to process it rather than bolt.

Veterans rarely walk in with only PTSD. Depression, anxiety, pain, and substance use often join them. Psilocybin-assisted therapy has already shown meaningful benefit for depression and anxiety when it is paired with careful preparation and integration. That matters in veteran care, where comorbidity is the norm and one stuck system can jam the rest. The VA is funding psychedelic work now, and some states and countries allow supervised psilocybin services. The federal status has not changed, so anything clinical lives inside research or regulated programs. That said, state programs are allowing psilocybin to be used in a therapeutic context and, as we noted before, some states have decriminalized it outright. Veteran mental health is an important issue on both sides of the aisle and anything that can improve outcomes is fast getting green-lit in Congress.

A typical PTSD psychedelic protocol is simple and demanding. You meet with therapists to set intentions and align expectations. You spend one or two full days in a safe room with eyeshades and music while two clinicians keep watch. You come back for multiple integration sessions to turn the experience into skills, insights, and behavior. Set and setting are vital. If the mindset is unrealistic, for example expecting a cure in a capsule, or the room is cold and clinical, outcomes suffer.

Psychedelic research has design headaches. It is hard to blind people to whether they got the medicine, which boosts expectancy and can inflate results. Veteran participation in the strongest MDMA PTSD trials has been limited, which means psilocybin PTSD trials need to recruit larger and more diverse veteran samples inside VA settings.

There are also practical hurdles. Many protocols ask people to taper SSRIs and other psychoactives before dosing, which is not trivial. Some medical conditions increase risk. Time is a real cost, and a single dosing day runs six to eight hours, and the prep and integration visits stack up. Providers need training, and two clinicians usually sit with the veteran during the experience, which ties up a clinic day for both.

Even with all of that, the treatment plan is straightforward. Trauma therapy asks you to approach what you avoid. Psilocybin can reduce avoidance and increase openness long enough to do the work. It is not a fix on its own, but it is a tool that, in the right hands, can help veterans turn toward what hurts and come back with something useful.

I asked Charlesworth what kind of veterans were best suited for mushroom therapy. She told me that they simply had to be ready to change. Unfortunately, some of her fellow veterans were too rigid or afraid to try the medicines.

"I've been really fortunate where I haven't experienced too many of those folks. And if somebody did have that attitude, they're not ready to sit. I would encourage them to come back when they were ready. Because I wouldn't force this on or push this on someone who wasn't actively ready to receive it," she said. "This is something that I feel calls to you and when it's time to use it and time to integrate it, it will be time. I fully believe in divine timing and if someone's fighting it and is brushing it off, I could give talking points and facts and figures and case studies and references all day long, but if someone's not ready to receive it, it's just going to go in one ear and out the other."

Global governments are slowly waking up to the promise of psychedelics. In the United States, for example, change is coming from a strange place: conservative red state Texas.

In 2021, House Bill 1802 told the Texas Health and Human Services Commission to team with Baylor College of Medicine and a veterans' hospital to study psilocybin for treatment-resistant PTSD in veterans. The law did not legalize psilocybin. It ordered a clinical trial, a full review of the science on MDMA, psilocybin, and ketamine, and regular progress reports.

From that mandate came Baylor's STARLIGHT study,[3] a state-funded clinical trial of psilocybin-assisted therapy for veterans with PTSD. It uses two dosing days with preparation and integration and clinician-rated PTSD as the main outcome. Baylor's IRB record for the study was created on February 21, 2025. This is research, not treatment on demand. The point is to produce data that can support federal review later. For a Texas veteran, it is a real, lawful path into care-quality research without leaving the state.

Former governor Rick Perry has become a key Republican voice for psychedelic research in Texas. He links his shift to the stories of veterans, including Marcus and Morgan Luttrell, who sought care in Mexico when options ran out at home. In June 2025, Texas backed FDA-directed ibogaine trials with a $50 million state investment.

"I have always been open to new knowledge. The same thing with criminal justice reform and in-state tuition, as a Republican, I have my beliefs, but I am willing to change them once looking at the data and science," he said in an interview in June 2025.[4]

Texas is also signaling that it will not wait for Washington to take the first step. The legislature has continued to fund and expand psychedelic research aimed at trauma in veterans and first responders. The newest tranche points at ibogaine, but the mechanism is the same. Create state-backed trials, stand up a clinical research network, and be ready to pivot when the FDA reschedules a compound. That playbook matters for psilocybin too.

Federal headwinds are real. In 2024, an FDA advisory panel advised against MDMA therapy for PTSD, and the FDA later declined approval. That decision does not touch psilocybin directly, but it raises the bar for trial design, masking, and safety monitoring that Texas studies will have to meet. The upside is that Texas wrote its laws to live inside the federal process, not to fight it. When the FDA asks for veteran-specific data, the state can point to its own trials and say, here is what we found.

But people need help. Some veterans go to Oregon or Colorado. Those states let adults take psilocybin in licensed centers with a trained facilitator present. It is not a prescription. It is supervised use. You book an intake, do prep calls, and spend a full day in a quiet room with eyeshades and music. You pay out of pocket. For many vets, cost is the first wall. Travel is the second.

Charlesworth does that now, in addition to her other work as an advocate and podcaster. She knows it works.

"I entered this work reluctantly. This was truly like my last hope. I was so determined to kill myself that I had a plan. And I didn't believe in God. I didn't believe in any sort of afterlife and I was completely against religion, which I still sort of am to some degree. But I was like, you know what? My son is worth it. I was just throwing all the spaghetti at the wall and seeing if this sticks. So I'll try it."

She recommends going to places where it is legal abroad. Jamaica has fully legal psilocybin. The Netherlands sells truffles that contain psilocybin. Mexico has retreats that work with psilocybin and other medicines. VETS and similar groups help with screening, funding, prep, and integration, and they steer people to vetted centers. The model is simple. Stabilize at home, fly in, do the work with support, fly back, and keep working with a coach or therapist. Families often notice the change first. Fewer blowups. More sleep. A little more room in the day.

Some enroll in research. A handful of VA and university teams are running psychedelic studies. Slots are limited. Screening is strict. People on multiple meds may have to taper, which is not easy. If you get in, it is no-cost care inside a protocol with real prep and real integration. It is also slow, because science is slow.

"I'm really proud of the VA for moving towards official studies on some of these things," said Charlesworth. "There's seven active studies going on across the VA right now, I think mostly on the East Coast working with MDMA. And in order to do better, I think that needs to go to all VAs. And I also think that psilocybin needs to be added to that list."

"I know these things take time and there's a lot of bureaucratic red tape, but these things need to be expanded to all of the VAs. There's really no excuse that it's only at seven of them when there's such a powerful resonating force of proof from the number of veterans organizations that are here, the number of voices."

Many former service members describe what Amber Capone, the cofounder of Veterans Exploring Treatment Solutions (VETS), once said about her husband Marcus, a Navy SEAL: "I think I was more afraid of losing him stateside after his service than I ever was during the time of war because I felt he just didn't care to be alive."

I spoke to Amber and Marcus during a time of heightened interest in PTSD and veterans. In about 2023, much of the conversation had changed from "drugs are bad" to "medicines are good" and veterans were beginning to explore new treatments. The couple, Marcus bearded and jovial, his wife long-haired and with a bright, broad smile, look like poster children for a post-deployment couple. It wasn't always that way.

"Our journey in the psychedelic world started in 2017," said Amber Capone. "My husband served thirteen years as a Navy SEAL and was medically retired in 2013. So for the four years following our transition back into civilian life, he sort of ran the gamut on Western approaches that were available to him through military medicine and then the VA. Everything pretty much included SSRIs and a host of other pharmaceuticals and talk therapy. And he was just getting more and more frustrated as these things weren't working or he would encounter undesired side effects. He was just really struggling with purpose and identity and feeling like completely alone in this new battle."

Again, the same story, repeated.

"We had spent the preceding thirteen years largely apart. So, we're also struggling as a couple. And as more as the years ticked by, I knew that suicide was something that he was struggling with and I was desperate to help. I couldn't. I basically decided that I was not going to be able to do this anymore. I was preparing to leave him. I thought of my kids and what that would mean for them and I was afraid that even if I could escape this hell, they would be stuck without a father for the rest of their lives."

When nothing else worked, Amber arranged for Marcus to travel outside the country in 2017 for a psychedelic intervention. He took ibogaine and DMT, two of the strongest compounds in the pharmacological cabinet. Overnight, the spiral stopped. The healing wasn't complete, no single session erases years of trauma, but as Amber put it, it was "a tourniquet to stop the bleeding our family was experiencing."

"He was reluctant. He was like a jock," she said. "He was a collegiate athlete. He didn't do drugs and didn't associate with people who did drugs. Our perception was that this was drugs. This was hippie, it was weird, but when you're desperate, you're willing to try anything."

That experience was the beginning of the nonprofit Amber and Marcus went on to found. VETS doesn't provide therapy itself. Instead, it raises funds so veterans can attend vetted retreat centers abroad, and it pairs that financial help with coaching before and after the sessions. By 2023, they had funded more than seven hundred veterans. Surveys of recipients showed that over 94 percent reported major improvements in their lives afterward.

VETS also pushes for research and policy change. They helped secure the first Texas legislation to fund psilocybin studies with veterans, pairing Baylor College of Medicine with the Houston VA. Their approach is built on three pillars: resources, research, and advocacy.

The Capones' story fits into a larger movement that has been slowly resurfacing after decades underground. In *Psychedelic Medicine*, author Richard Louis Miller interviewed researchers who described psilocybin as "a medicine, not a drug," especially in trials where it was given to people with treatment-resistant depression or end-of-life anxiety. Those same protocols are now being adapted for veterans, who often don't qualify for conventional studies because of multiple overlapping diagnoses: PTSD, TBI, depression, chronic pain.

Stanislav Grof, one of the early pioneers, spent years studying how psychedelic therapy helps people confront trauma. In *Realms of the Human Unconscious*, he documented cases where veterans and terminally ill patients, facing unbearable fear, were able to move through what he called the "death-rebirth experience."[5] The confrontation with fear itself was often the mechanism of healing. This happened repeatedly in the PTSD sufferers I met. So-called ego death allowed these soldiers to come back as civilians.

Even microdosing research, far less dramatic than flood-dose ibogaine or psilocybin therapy, has shown hints of value. Reports mention reduced PTSD triggers, stabilized mood, and greater capacity for healthy habits.

Every day, roughly twenty US veterans die by suicide. Amber Capone likes to point out the bitter irony: Many of the medications dispensed by the VA carry black-box warnings that they can increase suicidal thoughts. As she put it, "I've never been able to fully understand how we're fighting the veteran suicide epidemic with medications linked to suicide."

What VETS and allied researchers are building is not a miracle cure. Psilocybin, ibogaine, or MDMA do not erase the battlefield. What they seem to do is give space, a moment when the loop of hypervigilance and despair breaks, and the veteran can begin the hard work of living again.

"We certainly worry about word spreading too quickly or misinformation being spread in a very, very honorable community that this is some sort of panacea. It is absolutely not. It unlocks the ability to do very hard work," said Capone. "But someone going to a vetted safe retreat and knowing that you know they're receiving the therapy that has been sourced and dosed appropriately in a safe setting and they're supported with prep and integration coaching by professionals before, during, and after is absolutely critical to the overall success."

The Capones' project and Charlesworth's work show how desperate families, grassroots fundraising, and the slow return of psychedelic science are converging. If the state of Texas can legislate studies, perhaps others will follow. And if veterans, the most respected constituency in American politics, are the ones speaking up, the stigma may finally begin to lift.

And Charlesworth? How is she feeling now?

She's so much better, she reports.

"I'll give you a silly example, but it will articulate the point perfectly," she said. "The old version of Amy could not deal with anything without being explosive in anger because I just had no ability to regulate my emotions and deal with them. My son just dyed his hair black the other day and he got black hair dye all over the house towels. And I laughed about it. I'm like, what a goofball. That is not how I would have handled it two, three years ago. I would have been like, what the heck? I can't believe you got black dye all over this. It's ridiculous. The reactions are so different."

"I've seen my son go from being kind of afraid to tell me about something he's broken or damaged, whatever, to now he's like, it's no big deal," she said, smiling.

"It's no big deal," she repeated.

Blue Meanie

One night in late March, I stood outside on a soft spring evening talking with my friend Mike. We had just finished a middle-aged dad jam, guitar and piano, at the pizza place around the corner. That room felt like Brigadoon for wannabe rockers. I could play guitar, badly, with people who didn't mind us ruining their dinner. Most nights the place cleared out by 8:30, and we could play for an hour without too much shame.

We never had an audience, which was fine. I was just enjoying getting better at guitar.

After I started microdosing, my playing, or at least my focus, felt better. I was more social, and the old sense of dread I carried as a journalist had lifted. I wanted to have fun and talk about personal stuff like our lives and our trips. So, Mike and I were not talking about guitars. We were talking about what he saw at a sushi place.

He told me a plate of sashimi almost attacked him. He said it with a straight face, then laughed. That is Mike. During my heaviest growing phase, I had given him most of my stash, mostly because I couldn't use it all. He and his new girlfriend liked to chew a bit every few weekends and see where the night went. He told me the mushrooms had improved their relationship.

"We take a handful and just cuddle," he said. This is a guy who looks like he wouldn't cuddle at gunpoint.

"But what were those that you gave me last time?" he asked. He said the batch I gave him was strong.

"Usually, we'd take a few pieces and then go out and see how things went," he said. "This time we took a little and went out to eat. By the time the food came, the little waving cat clock was talking to me, and the food looked strange."

He explained that the sushi turned on him, appearing weird and alive. His girlfriend was near tears.

They paid, then stumbled into the street, aiming for home.

"What were those mushrooms called?" he asked.

They were Blue Meanies.

Blue Meanie is the common name for *Panaeolus cyanescens*, a deep blue–staining species. It was first recorded in Sri Lanka and now grows across warm, humid regions. It bruises deep blue when treated roughly. Many consider it much stronger than *Psilocybe cubensis*. Mike agreed.

"I was lucky to make it home," he said. He and his girlfriend went straight to bed and stared into space while the mushrooms did their work. They huddled, hugging each other as they rolled through what was probably a low-level ego death. They enjoyed it, after the fact, but damn. He didn't eat any more of that batch.

Blue Meanie stems are thin and shift from white to gray as they mature. The caps run from tan to off-white and can look a bit wavy, sometimes speckled. The blue stain shows up fast on stems and caps where handled and they turn blue to an almost comic degree.

That's not just online babble. According to a study performed[1] by two German researchers on mushrooms seized by customs, Blue Meanie contained about 2.5 percent psilocybin and 1.194 percent psilocin in twenty-five samples. This made them the strongest hallucinogenic mushrooms found so far, an impressive feat in a world that also contains Penis Envy, another strong strain.

The nickname itself traveled with two currents. First, the obvious: They turn blue when handled and they're extremely potent. Second, the cultural echo from 1968, when the Blue Meanies were the cartoon villains in the Beatles' Yellow Submarine. By the early 1970s, mushroom fans were calling *Panaeolus cyanescens* "Blue Meanies," a name that stuck in counterculture slang.

Australia is where the modern story really took off. In 1969, a surfer ferried news of Blue Meanies from Hawaii to Queensland and spread the spores. After heavy rains, he reported, the pasturelands flushed with these blue-staining mushrooms that local kids and merchants blended into "golden top" smoothies. The scene spread fast. Alongside *cubensis*, the slim, far more potent *Panaeolus*, gained a reputation under that Blue Meanie name.

From there, the current moved around the tropics. In Bali, islanders and tourists alike picked the same species right off cow and water buffalo dung. Restaurants quietly served "omelettes" made with them through the 1980s and 1990s. The mushroom's potency helped the legend travel as quickly as backpackers did, expanding the popularity of Blue Meanies through a global whisper campaign.

The Blue Meanies were my first successful grow in a new kind of bin from North Spore called the BOOMR BIN. The name obviously suggested that these things would boom if given enough nutrients and love. It was a lidded plastic box with large holes covered in micropore tape. There was a built-in fan at the back of the bin and a control system for humidity which allowed the shroomies to get enough moisture to thrive. I also built several tools to make things easier. The first thing I got was a remote power switch for the LED lamp. This allowed it to turn on and off after a few hours to simulate sunlight for the fast-growing shroomies. I also built a heat sensor that turned on the aquarium heating pad and an oxygen sensor to send fresh air into the bin. This last part was most important because during this grow my mushrooms began to exhibit the fuzzies.

Beginners often panic when they see a soft white layer creeping up the stems or sitting on the surface. It looks like mold. It is not. It's called the fuzzies. It is mycelium responding to poor air exchange. When carbon dioxide builds up, the mycelium keeps growing along the stem instead of putting energy into clean caps. Think of it as a signal for low oxygen, too much humidity, and not enough fresh air. The BOOMR box had just the fix: a little fan that you could turn on at various speeds to clear out the carbon dioxide while sending in fresh air.

I learned about the fuzzies the hard way with the Meanies, however. Early on I forgot to run the fan. For two days it all looked fine and then the bases grew a white beard. I thought the batch was lost but I got online to figure it out and learned about the fuzzies. By the next day, the fuzz had pulled back. Mushrooms like it moist and stuffy but, like us, they also need to breathe.

Unfortunately, at least according to my Reddit research, the fuzzies often gave off false signals, resulting in growers who dumped their bins just as their mushrooms were entering late adolescence. Because some mold also looks like fuzzies, inexperienced growers would simply take a picture, ask "Am I cooked?" in a forum or subreddit, and then just dump their grow before enough old mushroom hands could respond with advice. During one grow I almost felt that I got cobweb mold, a fuzzy-looking mold that could grow in inch-high patches on an otherwise clean substrate. I saw two of these patches during my grow, turned on the fan, and they retreated into the dirt, showing me that I wasn't infected, just negligent.

What's happening when mushrooms get fuzzies is surprisingly cool. Mushrooms and their mycelium breathe oxygen and give off CO_2. In a closed space, CO_2 sinks and pools near the surface and around the bases. The fungi can tell and when the air gets stale, the organism chooses survival over growth. It throws out fine aerial hyphae along the stems to reach up into the thin layer of better air. That is the "fuzz." Again, it's the same organism, just changing its form to chase a gas gradient. It would be as if we could grow and deploy a snorkel if we were stuck underwater, something I doubt any of us are able to do very quickly or efficiently given our current evolutionary speed.

High humidity makes the fuzzies look even worse. Water on the surface slows evaporation, so the boundary layer of air stays thick and still. The mycelium reads that stillness as a lack of exchange. Instead of building flat, confident caps, it keeps spinning out cottony growth to increase surface area. In good air, stems stay smooth and caps set. In stuffy air, stems wear sweaters.

How do you know if you've got a sick tub? If you want a quick field test, use your eyes. Even bright white fuzz that matches the mycelium and pulls back when conditions improve is a breathing issue. Off colors, sharp edges, or sour smells point to something else. Either way, the first question to ask is simple: Is the bin breathing? When the answer is yes, the beards vanish and the fruits remember what they were meant to do.

The Blue Meanie grow went ahead without a hitch. That said, the grow was surprisingly small, with only a few small jars of dried shroomies to show for my work. It was one of these jars that I gave to Mike and that apparently turned a sushi spot into a house of mirth.

Thinking about Mike's experience, I wanted to understand how mushrooms were reshaping relationships. Early in my own mushroom journey and before I began this book, I spoke to a woman who had returned from a retreat just outside the city with news that startled her husband. After a weekend of ceremonies and two deep psilocybin sessions, she told him she wanted an open marriage. The mushrooms, she explained, had shown her a path toward expanding her sexuality. She said she had been exploring threesomes and relationships with women, and the experience convinced her that honesty about those desires was necessary. For her, the medicine didn't just ease private wounds; it cracked open the container of her marriage.

That kind of story left me wondering: What exactly was happening here? Mushrooms were not just shifting moods or easing depression. They were changing the ways people loved, desired, and communicated. Mike told me his relationship had been transformed. He and his partner felt closer, more honest, even if one or two trips left them rattled.

For me, the changes were quieter but just as real. The mushrooms made me vulnerable in a way I hadn't been since my father died. I found myself crying again, often, not out of despair but out of release. That kind of emotional openness had been locked away for decades. I also suspected that the microdosing I had been experimenting with was playing a role. It wasn't dramatic, but over time it chipped away at old defenses and lightened the load I carried into my relationships.

Mushrooms didn't offer a single script. For some people, they broke bonds. For others, they deepened them. But in every case, I heard about, they were pushing relationships toward honesty, toward whatever version of intimacy the people involved had been too afraid to ask for before.

To get right down to it, micro- and macrodosing mushrooms is shown to be helpful with folks with low libidos. On the surface, this can mean something as simple as an increase in desire. Guides to microdosing list "enhanced sexual drive" among the most common benefits, alongside improved mood, energy, and creativity. People often describe their senses as heightened, touch more electric, colors brighter, and music richer, which can carry into intimacy.

But the effects run deeper than physiology. In therapeutic settings, psilocybin has been shown to lower defenses and soften the walls people build around themselves. One psychonaut, R. Coleman, wrote a book titled *Psychedelic Psychotherapy* that talked about his own journey through to better health and a healthier relationship.[2]

He wrote that these medicines dissolve fear and open the heart, making it possible to feel and express affection that had been buried under trauma. Couples who journey together sometimes speak of rediscovering each other, of feeling waves of empathy and compassion that remind them why they fell in love in the first place.

"As I continued psychedelic therapy, I discovered and worked through the trauma of childhood neglect and abuse," he wrote. "Hidden sources of my chronic illness, anxiety, and depression were revealed. My colitis healed, my depression vanished, and my health improved. As my sexual and relationship issues healed, I was able to manifest the healthy, happy marriage I enjoy today."

The cultural record points in the same direction. Andy Letcher, in his history *Shroom*, notes how mushrooms have long been linked to love, describing them as adding "sparkle into a loveless, synthetic world."[3] Across traditions, mushrooms are associated not just with visions and mysticism, but with the bonds that tie people together.

Taken together, the evidence suggests that mushrooms support intimacy in two ways. On one level, microdoses can boost libido and sharpen sensuality. On another, higher doses can open the emotional and spiritual channels that sustain long-term relationships. In both cases, they remind us that connection, whether physical or emotional, is at the core of healing.

Now, again, this is all woo-woo. The cynical journalist in me sees this kind of discussion as problematic because there is no way to identify "libido" or "sharpened sensuality" except, I suppose, when you snuggle on mushrooms. Countless club kids are still taking shroomies and ecstasy for decades and, although we didn't get a new Age of Aquarius, we could argue that much of EDM culture is definitely a lovefest.

That said, controlled studies point to some kind of change in people who use shroomies. Volunteers in psilocybin research frequently report feelings of emotional closeness and profound connection to others. In follow-ups, many say that the experience improved their ability to listen, to forgive, and to stay present in relationships. These effects can last well beyond the session itself, creating a sense of relational healing.

One study focused on libido and antidepressants. Titled "Psychedelics and Sexual Functioning: A Mixed-Methods Study"[4] and led by Tommaso Barba, it suggested psychedelic use, including psilocybin therapy, may improve some aspects of sexual functioning that SSRIs often worsen.

Selective serotonin reuptake inhibitors, the standard prescription for depression, are associated with sexual dysfunction in 40–65 percent of patients. As the authors note, "SD is therefore a risk factor for treatment adherence and resulting relapse or recurrence of a depressive episode." Against this backdrop, the team at Imperial College asked a simple question: What happens when you replace SSRIs with psilocybin?

The study combined two approaches. First, an online survey of over 1,400 people who used psychedelics in naturalistic or ceremonial settings. Second, a controlled clinical trial that randomized patients with major depression to either psilocybin-assisted therapy or six weeks of escitalopram, a.k.a. Lexapro, a popular antidepressant.

Across both groups, the results pointed in the same direction. Naturalistic users reported significant and lasting improvements in pleasure, appearance satisfaction, partner satisfaction, and sexual communication. They also described sex as more spiritual and felt greater openness to try new things. These changes held at both the four-week and six-month follow-ups. As the authors write, "participants . . . were more likely to perceive sex as a spiritual or sacred experience post-use."

The clinical trial reinforced these results. Patients treated with psilocybin, but not escitalopram, showed improvements in communication, partner satisfaction, sexual pleasure, and spirituality. The contrast was stark: "Patients receiving psilocybin were significantly more likely . . . to report higher, rather than lower levels of interest, arousal, activity, and satisfaction." By contrast, escitalopram patients often reported declines in those same domains, along with more anxiety around sex.

Now here's the rub: Like the woman I spoke to about her open marriage, it seems that when one partner tries mushrooms and the other doesn't, some interesting things happen, namely the desire for an open marriage. Shroomies seem to be tearing down traditional norms around relationships thanks to enhanced libido and everything associated with that.

The paper speculates that psychedelics' known capacity to increase mindfulness and connectedness plays a role. Traits like openness, non-judgment, and emotional presence map neatly onto what sex therapists describe as the components of "great sex": authenticity, communication, intimacy, and transcendence. The authors also note the possible role of attachment, citing evidence that psilocybin therapy reduces attachment insecurity, an issue tightly linked with sexual dissatisfaction.

The limitations of the study are real. Most survey participants were white, straight, and well-educated. The clinical sample was small. And as the authors caution, "our results should not be confused with 'drug-sex' or 'chem-sex.' . . . our focus has been on longer-term changes post–psychedelic use or psilocybin therapy."

Still, this is the first quantitative study to show what users have said for years: Psychedelics can improve sexual functioning and intimacy. The authors conclude, "psilocybin therapy . . . might be linked with improvements in sexual functioning. On the other hand, escitalopram . . . seemed to negatively impact sexual functioning."

So basically, what I was taking during my darkest hours was destroying my libido. Meanwhile, mushrooms were bringing it back. And I noticed. After hating on the gazelle people at the first mushroom events I went to, I came at further experiences with a far more open mind. While the group sessions never descended into orgies, I at least didn't mind hanging out with these folks anymore and found them pleasant and even attractive. Interestingly, one thing many facilitators say during longer mushroom retreats is to remind participants that they shouldn't have any sex with each other during their time at the event. They often found that sometimes when you took a few shrooms, even the most staid and controlled events slid into some kind of swingers' ball.

To understand this more, I spoke to Skye White, Skyler White on her birth certificate, though she doesn't like that name since the TV show *Breaking Bad* came out. Skye is a family and relationship therapist in San Diego who spent her formative years in rural, religious Arkansas, where she was told her feelings, her sexuality, and her kinks were bad.

Now Skye is much happier. She smiles as we talk, her face framed by chin-length dark hair, a nose ring in her left nostril. She works for the Affirming Therapy Center, a group of therapists that promise "our sex-positive therapists will partner with you to create a supportive, healing environment where you can feel safe to express your own truths while reorienting yourself toward joyfulness, playful curiosity, and loving connections."

Skye was joyful. Her first real clients were those same religious Arkansans: her parents.

"You know, I'm lucky. My family's always been open-minded, and my parents are pretty supportive," she said. "They don't always understand the things that I'm talking about, but I have, you know, been open with them, and my parents actually attended a music festival with me and have a memory of my mom and dad in a little cuddle puddle after they had taken MDMA."

"We were watching Diplo, and they were just giggly and cuddly, and it was adorable. And totally unexpected, you know, they're fairly straitlaced."

She began her own process of healing when she went to Arkansas State University at eighteen.

"I grew up in the meth capital of Arkansas. So, I knew there were certain drugs I never wanted to touch and didn't have any interest in going near. I started hanging out with more people that were dabbling in drugs that piqued my interest. I got more curious and felt a little trapped in that environment growing up.

"I was queer, I was poly, I was kinky, and not a lot of other people understood what that even was," she said.

"Psychedelics opened the door for me to explore my own identity in a way that didn't really require anybody else's input. And also, just kind of allowed me to accept those aspects of myself, you know, things that had always really kind of brought me a lot of shame and this sense of alienation."

She said that taking mushrooms was like five years of therapy in one night. She loved them and wanted to use them to help people.

When I asked White about how psychedelics influence intimacy, she paused before answering. "Clinically, people are kind of scared to talk about it," she said. "There's been so much misuse historically because there's no real quality control for facilitators. Psychedelics have been misused a lot in this regard."

She meant the weird, unregulated edge of psychedelic therapy, where trust and boundaries are sometimes broken. This edge is why many facilitators talk about sex at events. The mushrooms are potent medicine and not everyone can consent when using them, even after full sessions. Yet she believes that when done ethically, in a safe therapeutic context, these medicines can do something remarkable: "They can help bring down defenses. They can foster empathy. They can kind of interrupt communication patterns that people have been stuck in by resetting that default mode and allowing for shifts in perspective and a little bit more cognitive flexibility in relationships."

Skye has heard many of her clients describe unexpected effects on sexuality and self-image.

"It's all anecdotal," she cautioned, "but I've heard a lot of people talking about really positive impacts on self-image, which influences sexuality, and on their willingness and ability to engage and kind of pursue the kind of sex that feels satisfying or that they're excited to be having."

In her work, that often translates to people feeling more at home in their own bodies, more capable of closeness, and less bound by shame.

In the 1970s, Stanislav Grof saw something similar in his LSD-assisted psychotherapy sessions. He wrote that "sexual experiences and behavior can be deeply influenced by the LSD process. The intensity, depth, and completeness of the sexual orgasm and the ease with which it occurs seem to be closely related to the process of letting go of psychological defenses. . . . As LSD subjects learn to let go in the death-rebirth process, their orgasmic ability increases considerably; this improvement of sexual experiences can be observed in both males and females."[5]

He also observed that "Sexual neuroses, such as frigidity, vaginal spasms (vaginism), genital pain during intercourse, impotence, and premature ejaculation frequently respond well to LSD psychotherapy; however, effective treatment of these disorders usually requires serial administrations of the drug and experiential confrontation of the roots of these disorders on the perinatal level."[6]

Coleman described a related process: "When psychedelics open your heart, all the pain is still there, just as fresh and intense as the day you shut the door on it." Once the pain is felt and released, "the protective walls you built around your heart will melt. You will now be able to love and let love in deeply." They underline what Skye and Grof both describe: the return of connection.

Coleman also gives solid advice for folks looking to help their sexuality and relationships with psychedelics. He wrote:[7]

> At some points in your journeys, you may feel like you are going crazy. This most commonly happens on higher doses of psilocybin or LSD. Don't panic. The feeling of going crazy may also be part of remembering and releasing the confusion and unbearable pain that originally overwhelmed your mind.
>
> If you are experiencing craziness, focus your attention outside of the turmoil in your head. Stay centered in your body and your breath. As you feel and release the trauma, the craziness will eventually pass. This is a healing process. Let it happen.
>
> Your psychological and social development may have been impaired by childhood trauma. As you heal, you may need to learn skills from missed developmental stages. For example, if your wounds prevented you from healthy adolescent dating, you might now need to navigate this arena like a beginner.

In that sense, the psychedelic experience is not simply about sex at all, it's about intimacy, about recovering the capacity to give and receive love without the armoring of pain or expectation.

Today, therapists like White use the same language of safety and presence that Grof and Coleman did decades ago. She sees sexuality not as an isolated topic but as one expression of a person's ability to feel connected. "It's all tied to empathy and communication," she said. "When those open up, sex just changes too."

White also says that the medicine can help with the physical side of lovemaking.

"I've heard people talking about kind of like unlocking the ability to have multiple orgasms or kind of overcoming their gag reflex if they're having like psychedelic-assisted sex," she said. "But of course, it's not always positive. It can increase anxiety and cause performance issues. So there are two sides to every coin."

Interestingly, White has been working with people who are branching out and finding new ways to love. This came up again and again in the stories I heard, people who took one dose of mushrooms and realized they wanted more out of their relationships, or discovered they were no longer in love with their partners.

"We do a lot of identity exploration," said White. "The relationships that I work with tend to be people exploring non-monogamy. So, a lot of polyamory, swinging, open relationships, that kind of thing. And I do find that people that are engaging in more alternative lifestyles tend to also be called to find alternative methods for healing and therapy."

Skye is clear about what this work looks like when it is done with care. The point is not to chase a feeling. Instead, the point is to make room for better conversations, safer choices, and relationships that feel honest.

If you try this, treat it like the fragile thing it is. As Skye says, "Start slow, you know, you could always take more, you can't take less, and it's definitely better to dip your toes and kind of ease into the pool, than dive in headfirst and, you know, and traumatize yourself or have a bad experience." That is the ethic that runs through her practice.

Did mushrooms turn me into a sexual dynamo? Not really, but they did change the way I approached my relationships, including my marriage. Microdosing made me more patient, more gregarious, and a lot more joyful. It also reminded me that I was a sexual, and sexy, older man, and I tried to celebrate my body more. Your results may vary, obviously, but, like Mike, it might be worth testing the theory that mushrooms can make your relationships better even if they occasionally make your sushi talk to you.

Illusion Weaver

It was a crisp fall day and I was in a rental house in the middle of the woods. I was with three friends I wanted to introduce to mushrooms, so, like a diligent psychonaut, I took care with set and setting. I meted out a dose of Illusion Weaver, a strain I had grown on a whim after seeing it in a spore catalog.

Illusion Weaver sits in the family of named *Psilocybe cubensis* varieties that move through spore forums and vendor catalogs. Many sellers compare it to Golden Teacher because of the small golden caps and approachable growth, but that is a visual and cultural comparison, not a proven lineage. Descriptions often mention long, slightly twisty stems and small caramel-to-golden caps that can show faint veining at maturity. Some of them have a little white cap at the top, a fluffy bit of mycelium that is rare in other types. The "weaver" idea probably comes from that look. It is treated as a domesticated, designer line rather than a wild type. Origin stories usually point to selective work by underground growers. Some accounts credit a Florida collector who found it and grew it and then passed it on to a seller known as the Keeper. None of that is documented in a way a scientist would accept, but we're not scientists, are we?

Reputation and effects live in the marketing copy. Illusion Weaver gets pitched as visual-forward and strong for a *cubensis*. Treat that as anecdotal. Within *P. cubensis*, set, setting, dose, and grow conditions shape chemistry more than the sticker on the bag. Genomics for these named varieties are rarely standardized, and even the same label can drift over time as growers clone and reclone standout fruits.

It was sunny and warm inside. I put out small snacks and set up a large speaker, then connected it to my phone. I built a playlist, basically something I found while searching for "psychedelic trip playlist," and added a few favorites. "This Bitter Earth" sung by Dinah Washington and remixed by Max Richter. Some Grant Green guitar jazz. I added "River" by Leon Bridges at the end, right where I liked it during trips with the group back home. Tripping playlists are an art. I wasn't great at them, but because nearly everything sounds good on mushrooms, I figured I could pull it off.

All three of us settled into our nooks. One friend, Matt, took the lounger. Another friend, Rob, stretched out on a ratty couch. I made a little nest out of blankets on the floor and lay back, ready to celebrate the magic of the shroom.

The trip set in quickly, and fractal images poured through the skylight above me. On the couch, Rob smiled. Matt wandered around the house, staring at kitchen appliances. I should have told him to sit still, but he wanted to explore.

Meanwhile, I was thinking about my father.

He had been a big man, nearly 375 pounds in his prime. Big in the way folks were big in the 1970s, tall, imposing, huge hands, a chest and belly that didn't sag so much as form a solid mix of fat and muscle. His body was born of beer, tamales out of a jar, and a sedentary life led at the Defense Construction Supply Center in Columbus and then, when he retired with a military pension, the floor in front of our big old TV set.

I missed him. I missed his scent, something like sweat and grease. We would listen to NPR in the garage while we changed the oil in his VW Vanagon or did the brakes on my Ford Fairmont station wagon, the car I got when I turned sixteen. I thought about how I used that old station wagon to build sets for high school plays. We would load it with plywood and paint and drive it back to school, a few friends sitting, unbelted, in the back. He had made that happen, indirectly. He helped me form my first lasting friendships with folks I still know and love today.

I smelled him. I smelled the plywood. I smelled the oil from the VW and the anti-seize he would dollop onto tire lugs, explaining that a little thread grease now kept the whole thing from locking up later.

I saw his bottle of Molson Ice near his right hand, always ready. I smelled his cigars.

I saw his old workbench. He had bolted a beautiful American-made vise to it when I was one or two, and he used it to pull parts apart or glue things together. The bench was covered with jars full of nails and screws, all laid out in an organizational system that baffled everyone except him. He had skeins of old telephone wire, endless spare parts for our old cars, and a beer fridge that smelled, inexplicably, like the Whatchamacallit candy bars he once kept in there.

I got all that from that trip. Near the peak, when my metabolism had taken in all the psilocybin it could, I heard his voice.

"Be a better father," he said.

I joked back at him. What did he know about that?

It wasn't all thread grease and love. He had been mean. Nasty, even. He turned into a Rush Limbaugh Republican and then a Trumper. He did it because Limbaugh and Trump reminded him of the guys at work, the people who let him make racist and sexist jokes on company time, the guys he used to drink with. He told horrible, racist jokes to his hospice nurses. He spent his time cursing out people who posted things wrong on Craigslist. He was selfish and oafish and loud and had been a mean drunk when we were kids. There was a period, some kind of strange fugue, when he would beat my mother after work, yelling at her for something I didn't understand. He was a bad father.

But wasn't I just like him? I was a grumpy drunk, a political changeling who could be cruel and crass. I listened to my own brand of brainwashing, my own Fox News, in the form of endless doomscrolling and echo-chamber news. I told myself I was left of him, more educated, with better jobs. He was, I sneered, a paper pusher. I thought that made me a better man.

But was I?

Absolutely not. We were the same.

"Be a better father."

He said it again, as clearly as if he were in the room. I was wide awake. His voice came through the sunlight.

He did not say it as an admonition. He said it as a warning. He did not mean I needed to be a better father right now. He meant I had to be a better father than he was.

That is when I learned that mushrooms could connect us to the past and soften grief. Even with that dark message, I heard him and saw him and smelled him and was with him for a moment.

I was comforted by the presence of the man who once taught me to read, to love Shakespeare, to laugh uproariously at Monty Python, to tell a joke and crack a beer and be the life of the party.

That other dad, the one who wheeled around in his chair and embarrassed me when he took too much of everything and insulted the waiters at the Chinese buffet on Morse Road, was gone, replaced by sunlight.

And I could forgive him.

Using mushrooms in this way, to solve big head problems, isn't new. In fact, it's become the de facto use case for most clinicians exploring psychedelic therapy. Taking a few grams, four to six, usually, and lying around thinking has become the new therapy for countless people in pain. I wanted to explore a few ways people were using mushrooms the way I did and how they used them when all hope was lost.

The true spiritual value of shroomies shouldn't be discounted. Mushrooms, as we learned before, have had a long history in religious worship and have especially been considered a gateway into other dimensions and spiritual realms. While I consider that mostly hokum, there was an interesting study that pointed to the value of mushrooms when it came to internal growth and self-love.

One of the most striking examples of this happened on Good Friday, 1962. In the basement of Marsh Chapel at Boston University, Harvard divinity student Walter Pahnke gave psilocybin to ten theology students. Upstairs, a crucifixion sermon ran through the chapel speakers. Downstairs, something else took shape. The students who got the drug reported classic mystical states and later ranked the session among the most meaningful experiences of their lives. One tried to leave the chapel to preach his revelation in the streets of Boston and had to be held back. The Good Friday Experiment became a touchstone for modern research on psychedelics and religion.

Pahnke's question was old and blunt: Can you reliably bring on the kind of experience people describe as divine? Working with Timothy Leary, he set the session in a church and used William James's checklist for mystical experience. This included unity, a sense that time and space have dropped away, and a difficulty putting the experience into words. Pahnke tried to measure what most traditions have only pointed to.

You can hear the echo from older rites. For example, the Greeks held the Eleusinian Mysteries, where initiates drank something called kykeon and saw the afterlife. Some scholars think ergot was involved. Others, like Wasson, argued that mushrooms were the hidden sacrament.

The mushrooms truly helped when I hit a bad patch around age forty-eight. My oldest son had just gone off to college and left a huge hole in the house. While he was distant in middle school, he became a real buddy in high school and watching a sullen boy turn into a tall, capable young man was thrilling. Then he left.

The change blasted a hole in our lives and although friends told me that he was doing exactly what kids were supposed to do when they wandered off into the world, my attachment was still strong. I hit another depression; this one coupled with anxiety.

I started the microdosing around this time and chose Illusion Weaver, the mushroom that let me talk to my dad, as the first one to try. Illusion Weaver was one of the more esoteric mushrooms I grew.

The strain felt more modern than anything else I had grown, including JMF, so I gave it a go. The name hinted at secret knowledge, which did not hurt, but again, mushroom names are mostly bluster.

Illusion Weaver, for me, became an example of how naming, lore, and aesthetics fused into the modern *cubensis* scene. Small communities name a mushroom based on how it looks and a story forms on forums. Vendors repeat the story and a brand is born. None of that makes the experiences fake but it does mean we should keep the categories straight and not expect too much out of individual types. Again, varieties like this are cultural and, in their own way, they make folks think that they've got something special and different when it comes to their latest varietal. Unlike apple or tomato varieties, the names often tell more about the grower than the fruit.

Enough about varietals. Back to the priests tripping in a basement. The original Good Friday study had problems. It was a small sample with imperfect controls. Yet it opened a lane that later teams would drive down.

In October 2015, Roland Griffiths, William Richards, and Anthony Bossis set about doing it again. This time they used modern screening and clinical support. They were looking for religious leaders who wanted to deepen their spiritual lives through a supervised psilocybin session.[1]

First, a bit about the psychonautical pedigree exhibited here. Roland R. Griffiths was an American psychopharmacologist who helped bring psychedelic research back into top-tier medicine. He earned his PhD in psychopharmacology at the University of Minnesota in 1972, then joined Johns Hopkins, where he became a professor of psychiatry and behavioral sciences and neuroscience. Early on, he defined caffeine dependence and withdrawal in careful human studies, work that shaped clinical guidance on a drug most of us use daily. In 1999 he turned to classic psychedelics. His 2006 paper showing that psilocybin can occasion "mystical-type" experiences with lasting personal meaning became a pivot point. That work, and follow-ons, set the stage for trials in depression, addiction, and cancer-related distress. In 2019, Hopkins launched the Center for Psychedelic and Consciousness Research, with Griffiths as founding director.

He was not above debate. In 2024, reporting surfaced on a complaint by longtime colleague Matthew W. Johnson that criticized aspects of the lab's methods and framing, prompting wider scrutiny of setting, expectancy, and interpretation. The discussion continues across journals and media, a sign of a field still testing its claims in public.

The team also included William Richards, another central figure in the modern revival of psychedelic research. Richards came to the field after a powerful meditation experience that pushed him past a purely material view of the mind. His group, alongside Griffiths's, ran clinical work showing psilocybin could relieve fear and anxiety in cancer patients. That 2016 study became a landmark and helped open the door to many trials with psilocybin and MDMA.[2]

The design was randomized, double blind, cross-over, with two dosing days about five weeks apart. Each person received a very low dose in one session and a high dose in the other, both with the same therapy, preparation, and integration. The team used standard clinician ratings and self-reports. They measured mood, anxiety, quality of life, sense of meaning, optimism, and fear of death at five weeks and again about six months later.

The results were striking. About two-thirds to four-fifths met criteria for a clinically significant drop in depression and anxiety after the high dose, and most held those gains at six months. People also reported better life satisfaction, more purpose, and less fear around dying. Adverse effects were mostly short lived, like nausea, headache, and brief blood pressure spikes, with no signal of new addiction or lasting harm. In plain terms, one high-dose psilocybin session, done with careful support, produced large and lasting relief for many of these patients.

But in 2012, Richards and NYU psychologist Anthony Bossis had started asking how psychedelics intersect with religion. Could a properly supported session help clergy with well-being, vocation, and faith? Would it deepen their tradition or shake it? Philanthropists helped fund the work. Some later took roles as interviewers or session facilitators.

A few spiritual folks joined the study, including a Catholic priest, a Baptist biblical scholar, several rabbis, an Islamic leader, and a Zen roshi. Four were Episcopalians. The sample skewed white and male. Recruiting across some traditions proved difficult, in part because of prohibitions against intoxicants. Finding rabbis was easy. Finding rabbis without prior psychedelic experience was harder.

The study had clear limits. First, there was the small sample size and tendency toward self-selection. There was also no placebo control and an expectancy effect, essentially the idea that the clergy were looking forward to the trip, was likely. Language and music choices leaned Christian, which some participants noticed. Still, as a window into a rare population, it produced detailed accounts of high-dose sessions among clergy. Most reported lasting shifts in prayer, vocation, and their sense of the sacred. A large majority ranked the experience among the most meaningful of their lives.

The session followed the modern protocol. It included several prep meetings and then took place in a comfortable room with a couch. Participants wore headphones and an eye mask. Two trained guides led each participant through the experience. Their reports were similar: These participants from different faiths called the sessions among the most meaningful of their lives. Some said it deepened their tradition. Others felt a loosening of strict boundaries and a glimpse of a shared core.

In a piece by Michael Pollan in the *New Yorker*,[3] each of the participants described experiences that seemed to mimic the traditional style of religious ecstasy. The Muslim representative, a British woman named Sughra Ahmed, said that she was "petrified" at first but then felt a deep connection to Allah as the trip progressed:

> Early in her first session, Ahmed told me, she felt God right behind her. "Like, if I turned around, I would bump into God,"

> she said. "There's a verse in the Quran in which God says, 'I'm closer to you than your jugular vein.' The jugular is the life-giving source. God was with me the whole time." For her, God was neither masculine nor feminine. "God was above gender, above everything . . . an existence, not a figure," she said. "And God was love." Her epiphany was a familiar psychedelic trope, but that did not make it any less profound. "It was just mind-blowingly clear how wrong we have it as human beings, and how we need to nurture love, to put it at the center of our engagement with humanity and animals and the planet," she told me.

Another member of the clergy, a minister at Emmanuel Episcopal Church on Mercer Island in Washington, described it as the laying on of hands. "It blew out of the top of my head, and then I started making these sounds that felt religious and spiritual and sacred," the priest, named Hugh Priest, said. "I realized I was speaking in tongues, which I had never done before. Speaking in tongues is not an Episcopal sort of thing."

Not everyone felt clarity. A Protestant minister said nothing about his session felt specifically Christian while a Buddhist roshi found it deeply nonconceptual and hard to describe. Rita Powell, now the Episcopal chaplain at Harvard, met the abyss and declined a second session. She later said the preparation did not cover how dark it could get.

The paper reported that participants often described authentic religious experiences and a felt presence rather than a visible deity. Several encountered symbols outside their own tradition. Many met the divine in a feminine register and spoke of God as soothing or maternal. Some described a deconstruction of patriarchal religion. Many reported a new appreciation for other faiths and a softer grip on rigid doctrines. A few admitted less tolerance for institutional forms of worship and the tension between orthodoxy and direct experience was on full display.

Other stories focused on renewal in ministry. An Eastern Orthodox priest described a death-rebirth vision in the tomb of Christ and a decisive softening of anger and burnout. He spoke of recovering love for the liturgy and a more open heart. Hugh Priest said the experience simply made him a better pastor and delayed his retirement. Several argued that clergy should be prepared to help parishioners integrate psychedelic experiences, regardless of legal status.

Taken together, the stories point to a simple claim: Psychedelics resemble spiritual awakening more than mental illness. Many of the clergy, perhaps not the Buddhist, did not see themselves as mystics. The sessions changed that. Mushrooms opened them to experiences they called sacred.

The work raised questions about conflicts and bias. A Johns Hopkins IRB audit found reporting problems and unapproved roles for a funder and a registered researcher who was also a funder. The board notified the FDA and required disclosures. Senior researchers acknowledged the issues and said donors should not conduct research activities while others worried about public perception and possible backlash from organized religion.

Hunt Priest took the biggest step. He left parish work and went on to found Ligare, a Christian psychedelic society that frames psilocybin as a potential sacrament of grace. The group has hosted retreats in the Netherlands and now Priest argues that churches can offer safe containers and centuries of wisdom on ritual, ethics, and community. He also says the psychedelic world can learn from religious traditions about care, humility, and integration.

Nearly a decade after dosing began, the clergy study sits in a charged place. It shows the promise and the risks. It shows how a single session can deepen compassion, loosen rigid beliefs, and widen respect for other paths. It also shows how preparation, cultural fit, and integration affect outcomes. Whether this becomes a bridge between institutions and direct experience, or a new front in an old fight, remains open.

For the participants, the lasting thread is simple. A carefully held session gave them a vivid sense of the sacred. Some called it God.

Some called it unity. Many walked back into their ministries with a different heart.

Stanislav Grof has described these sessions as initiations as much as therapies. In *The Way of the Psychonaut*, he writes about holotropic states that mirror shamanic trance and religious ecstasy.[4] People report archetypal scenes, powerful symbols, and at times a clean sense of union. The pattern often looks like death and rebirth, which you can also find in baptism, in the Tibetan Book of the Dead, and in other traditions that teach people how to die before they die.

What surprised people in the clergy study was not only the intensity of what happened but the aftershocks. Participants talked about renewed compassion, a broader curiosity about other faiths, and a softer hold on rigid ideas. One rabbi said he was flooded with love.

This is where the modern meets the old. In *Storming Heaven*, Jay Stevens traces how LSD and psilocybin moved from labs to living rooms in the 1960s, often framed as a new sacrament for a new spirituality.[5] Timothy Leary spoke in that register for years. Today's researchers are more careful. They talk about set and setting, screening, integration, and the limits of small studies while avoiding mention of the spiritual. All of that is for the participants to find.

These studies, as esoteric as they were, began to connect two disciplines: hospice care and psychedelic facilitation. Mushrooms, integrators felt, could help reduce the fear of loss, of decline, of dying, yes, but also decrease the fear of looking foolish, of being vulnerable again after a lifetime of holding it together. Boomers are becoming more integrated with the shroomies and their goals are simple: to approach the end of life with grace and to eat more mushrooms.

Josh, a trained psychedelic facilitator whose partner is a hospice nurse, sees this change up close. "There's a real concern among older folks about dying," he told me. "They want comfort, ease, clarity. But most don't plan for it. They don't talk about it. And that's where psychedelics can open a window."

His work isn't medical, and it isn't evangelical.

"I don't try to bring anything out of the experience," he said. "I'm there to hold space. For someone facing a terminal diagnosis, that might mean half a gram of mushrooms. For others, just sitting in silence, talking about breath, tension, and legacy."

Late in life, after a diagnosis of metastatic colon cancer, Roland Griffiths himself spoke openly about mortality and his own carefully guided sessions. A widely read *New York Times* Magazine interview captured his thinking, and Hopkins profiled his reflections on gratitude and end-of-life awareness. He died on October 16, 2023.[6]

In his seminal final interview, Griffiths told us basically how he prepared to go:

> After getting the diagnosis, I had no immediate interest in psychedelics. I felt in many respects that I was having a very psychedelic-like experience. There was this awakening, this aliveness, and I hesitated to take a psychedelic because I wondered whether it was going to disrupt that. Then a question arose: Is there something I'm avoiding by not taking a psychedelic? Am I defending against some dark, fearful thing I'm in denial about? Am I papering it over with this story of how great I'm doing and actually I'm scared to death?

Josh's goal as a facilitator isn't to chase visions or heroic doses. It's about access, gentle, intentional access to emotions and insights that often stay buried. Sometimes that starts with ketamine.

"It helps people relax," Josh said. "It's short-acting, safe, and can take the edge off the fear spiral. Then we can begin to think about mushrooms or even 5-MeO."

For many in this cohort, boomers and older Gen Xers, it's not their first contact. "I hear this all the time," Josh said. "'I took mushrooms in college and had this wild experience. Haven't touched them since.' They're curious again. But now, instead of a dorm party, they want peace. They want to talk to their body. They want to feel something before they leave."

It's not a trip. It's a process.

Sometimes the work is as simple as noticing physical tension and asking, "What would your life feel like without this pain in your neck?" That small invitation becomes a doorway. From there, somatic work, breath, and guided meditation help create a container for change, whether medicine is involved or not.

And the stigma against drugs? It's real, but it's changing.

Josh offers no pressure.

"People are ready when they're ready," he said. "It took me years to trust MDMA and ketamine because of what I'd heard growing up. But language matters. I don't call it a drug. I call it medicine. The doctor gives you medicine to help you heal."

He told me about one man, tense, withdrawn, depressed for years, who came in with major treatment-resistant depression and walked out, after several sessions and a mushroom experience, with less fear.

"He wasn't suddenly 'happy,'" Josh said. "But his body was softer. His words had space in them."

This isn't about silver bullets. It's about presence. And it's about reminding people that they're allowed to feel curious again, even at the end.

Josh smiled as he shared a story about a woman visiting a nursing home in California, quietly offering low-dose 5-MeO to elders who couldn't leave their beds.

"She comes in and says, 'It's time for your medicine. Do you want it today?' And if the answer's no, she just comes back next week."

As we said before, shroomies are useful for palliative care. In an open-label trial at Sheppard Pratt in Baltimore, led by Scott Aaronson and published in the *American Journal of Psychiatry* in 2025, adults in a current major depressive episode with severe treatment-resistant depression, at least five failed treatments, received a single 25 mg dose of synthetic psilocybin.[7] They stopped psychotropic meds at least two weeks before dosing and for at least three weeks after, something that could have been quite trying for the subjects. The primary outcome was change on the Montgomery-Åsberg Depression Rating Scale, a standard scale for depression.

Depression scores fell sharply by week three and stayed lower at week twelve. In exploratory work, greater "oceanic boundlessness" during the session tracked with better antidepressant response. Participants with PTSD showed a weaker effect but the team reported the treatment as safe and tolerable in this setting.

This matters for the end of life, because depression and meaning are tied together when time is short. "Journeys are microcosms for life" is how psychedelic facilitator Livi Joy described her work with hospice patients. For her, it starts with armor. "Is it safe to take that armor off and really relax and allow whatever is under the surface to come up?" she asked. Her preparation work is built around that question, trust and letting go. "There's a switch that has to happen when the person is like 'I can trust this person to take care of me.'"

She prefers to meet people where they live. "When I work with folks one on one, I usually like to work in their space. It takes stress out of it. Ultimately, the place where people want to relax is in their home."

The session then becomes practice for what comes next. "Journeys are microcosms for life," she said. "Whether it's asking for help or a big emotion coming up and allowing it, it is practice for the rest of life." That practice often means learning to be held. "You need anything, please just ask," she tells clients, and hears the same reply. "It's really hard to ask for help." In session, that pattern can crack. "I can't stand up by myself," someone may admit. For hospice teams, that shift is the point. You rehearse receiving care and prepare for inevitable decline.

Her screening lens is blunt about timing and safety.

"I liken this work to shaking the snow globe," she said. "We want all of it to come up and see what we've been tripping over. But if the house isn't glued down well enough and you shake the snow globe, no bueno."

Translation for end of life is simple. The care environment must be stable and there has to be real time for integration. "Time and space to actually process the event" is "paramount," she said. "If you are a high-performing type A and you are just squeezing this in on a Saturday and going right back into it Sunday night, that might not be the best time."

The goal is to let the patient hand off control without feeling abandoned.

"I show them where all the things are in my home that they might need. Then I actually ask them to relinquish that and let me be the one taking care of you."

In microdosing language, it means using the medicine to help take some of the burrs off of your brain. It worked for me and I can only imagine what it would do for folks who are truly in distress.

Joy described her job as creating a clean handoff from autonomy to supported surrender. She watches for signs that standard coping has stalled and works with patients to help them understand what is happening and where they are going.

What Joy describes, and what I experienced, is the removal of armor. She means the armor of life, the armor we put on early in life that we wear to keep ourselves together, sane, and fed. It's armor that we wear with honor for decades until it's time to take it off, to become vulnerable.

"Create the environment for lasting meaningful change." In hospice, that is the work. She helps a person feel held and helps the family practice asking and receiving. She helps everyone name what is rising, then helps them carry it together.

It's this vulnerability that meant the most to me in all my mushroom experience, a way of dropping defenses and letting things just be. The cynic in me cringes at this but, thanks to people like Joy, I was able to finally take off that helmet of discomfort and, at times, anger.

Wavy Caps

When I spotted Wavy Caps on one of the spore sites I realized this was my next grow. After a few sci-fi and erotically themed shroomies it was nice to return to something that sounded like a gang of street urchins who wanted to beat up Peter Pan.

Psilocybe cyanescens, also called Wavy Caps, live where people stack wood and rake leaves. It thrives on lignin-rich landscaping debris, especially alder and mixed hardwood chips, and it tends to show up when autumn turns cold and wet. Caps start caramel to chestnut when moist, then fade to pale buff as they dry. At maturity the margins ripple into the namesake wave. Most tissues bruise deep blue when handled, which fits the name *cyanescens*, and the species sits close to several other wood-loving *Psilocybe*.

The Wavy Cap, *Psilocybe cyanescens*, entered the formal scientific record in 1946 when Elsie Maud Wakefield described it in Transactions of the British Mycological Society from specimens collected at Kew Gardens.[1] Wakefield did not "discover" the mushroom in the modern sense, but she provided the first valid taxonomic description and established the type locality at Kew. If sacred mushrooms have a quiet architect in the archives, it is Wakefield. A British mycologist, she joined the Royal Botanic Gardens, Kew, in 1910, became Head of Mycology in 1915, and later served as Deputy Keeper of the

Herbarium. Over the course of her career, she published close to a hundred scientific papers and produced careful illustrations to accompany her taxonomic work, at a time when line drawings were central to species identification.

By the time she published *Psilocybe cyanescens* in 1946, Wakefield had spent decades working on fungal systematics at Kew. The type specimen came from the gardens, which is why Kew remains listed as the type locality in modern references. Her description was part of a broader program of careful documentation of British fungi, many of them small brown wood-inhabiting species that are difficult to distinguish without close study. Wakefield's influence extended well beyond a single mushroom. She helped shape British mycology in the first half of the twentieth century and trained younger taxonomists who continued that institutional tradition.

Back in the mulch, the practical details return. Wavy Cap gills are attached to the stem and shift from light brown to dark purplish brown as spores mature. The odor and taste are "like the smell of freshly cut green beans and of flour," at least according to the Beaty Biodiversity Museum.[2] I could not corroborate that, since most specimens smelled simply mushroomy to me. In the Pacific Northwest and across temperate Europe, you find Wavy Caps in the same mulched beds that host other chip-lovers, often around Halloween. Under the scope, spores are smooth and elliptical, about 9 to 12 by 5 to 8 micrometers. That narrow range matters. It helps separate *cyanescens* from similar brown-capped, wood-chip species.

I grew them because I wanted to try *cyanescens*, a family of shroomies that is particularly blue and particularly intense.

This bluing is the reason this species built a reputation. *Psilocybe cyanescens* typically tests higher in tryptamines than many other *Psilocybe* species, and users report strong visuals, fast shifts in mood and thought, and a heavy sense of connectedness. But you must be careful foraging them in the wild, where they're often plentiful. In mixed urban beds, Wavy Caps can fruit in dense numbers that invite mistakes with toxic lookalikes, so you better know what you're doing.

Better yet, do what I did and don't pick them at all and instead grow them yourself.

By the time I started growing Wavy Caps, I had become the shroom guru to the parents and friends I talked to about the project. One friend, recently widowed, wanted some to make evenings a little more bearable. Another asked for a batch to microdose, and I even made her travel chocolates. The result of that experiment was a tray of very moist, very messy chocolate bears that looked a bit diseased, in which the ground-up mushrooms refused to stay coated.

People immediately asked me if they could pay me, whether I had advice on dosing, and what I thought was a good microdosing schedule. Not wanting to go to jail or offer incorrect advice, I was careful: No, you can't pay. That was a no-brainer. First, I wanted to be Johnny Mushroomseed and spread the magic of shroomies to all my middle-aged friends. Second, I didn't want to go to federal prison.

As for the dosing, I repeated what most online sources said about taking mushrooms, not realizing how variable potency can be: Take three grams at first and more if you don't feel anything, maxing out at five. About .15 grams a day was normal but dried mushrooms could vary in potency. The rule of thumb is that a stem is the same as a cap is the same as a small, unidentified lump of mushroom, but in reality one .15 dose could be a bit more effective than another.

All this information was basic and could be found online and in books. But I had it readily at my fingertips, and because I had a trove of shroomies I had to get rid of, I became vaguely more popular with a certain kind of adult: countercultural, dissatisfied with booze and pills, and willing to try anything just to smile again. Kind of like me in 2021 or so.

Being a glutton for punishment, I mused about building my own psychedelic practice or mushroom factory. All signs, however, pointed to "No."

In the early 2020s, mushrooms looked like a gold rush. Newly public psychedelic biotechs and glossy "functional mushroom" brands promised to reinvent mental health and wellness, then ran straight into multiple brick walls. Unlike ketamine, mushrooms were still federally illegal but, as we noted before, surprisingly easy to grow. Unlike cannabis, mushrooms also weren't a daily habit for many, resulting in lower demand over time. In other words, mushrooms weren't a cash crop simply because people took them very rarely and under controlled conditions. You don't do a mushroom trip like you go on a beer bender.

Regulation moved slower than Silicon Valley and the investors who might have loved taking shrooms in some Burning Man orgy tent were timid when it came to dumping money into start-ups promising limited returns on a product that grew naturally in mulch. Clinical timelines stretched. Retail hype cooled. By late 2025 you could see the pattern: A handful of drug developers with deep pipelines were still standing and they would probably come to market with Ashruminox or some similarly named medicine promising some of psilocybin's benefits without any of the fun. With the big guys firmly entrenched in research, many consumer plays had pivoted, paused, or disappeared.

The bellwethers went first. Compass Pathways, a company dedicated to turning mushrooms into medicine, listed on the Nasdaq in September 2020 and pushed psilocybin therapy into late-stage trials. In June 2025 the company reported its first Phase 3 success in treatment-resistant depression, a rare bright spot in a tough market. Compass CEO Kabir Nath saw a future catering to the Make America Healthy Again crowd, a strange amalgamation of the political left and right who were in search of alternatives to Western medicine. In fact, as we noted before, many conservative figures have come out in favor of mushrooms, especially for veterans and other sufferers of depression and PTSD.

"What's in the public domain is that both RFK Jr. and Secretary Collins have talked about trying to find a way to make psychedelics available within 12 months,"[3] said Kabir in August 2025, a year after the FDA refused to give Lykos Therapeutics a license to study midomafetamine (MDMA)-assisted therapy for PTSD. These moves dampened Compass' efforts and left the company stock deflated to about six dollars after an all-time-high of $59 in December 2020.

Atai Life Sciences followed with its own splash in June 2021, listing on Nasdaq during the height of the psychedelic investment boom. The company positioned itself less as a single-drug start-up and more as a holding company for psychedelic and adjacent therapies, building a portfolio that included compounds based on psilocybin, DMT, and other novel molecules. Like much of biotech, its stock has ridden a volatile path through the broader market downturn.

Rather than buying companies outright, Atai has tended to take large strategic stakes. In 2024 it became the largest shareholder in Beckley Psytech, a London-based drug developer founded by Lady Amanda Feilding and her son Cosmo Feilding Mellen. Beckley grew out of the Beckley Foundation, the research nonprofit Feilding created in the late 1990s to bring psychedelic science back into respectable laboratories.

Lady Amanda Feilding, who passed away in May 2025, was known popularly as the countess who drilled a hole in her head.

"Ms. Feilding, who was known as Lady Mindbender and the Crackpot Countess, once drilled a tiny hole in her skull to increase blood flow, a medieval practice called trepanning," said her *New York Times* obituary. "She believed that psychedelic drugs could be used to treat depression and other maladies, now a promising area of scientific study."[4]

Thankfully, she was also among the modern figures who helped pull psychedelics out of the counterculture and back into serious research. A real British countess, artist, and self-taught scientist, she founded the Beckley Foundation in 1998 to fund and advocate for psychedelic research at a time when almost no one else would touch it. Operating from her family estate at Beckley Park in Oxfordshire, she built quiet alliances with neuroscientists and policymakers to reintroduce LSD, psilocybin, and other compounds into legitimate study.

Feilding's approach mixed aristocratic patience with political pragmatism. She coauthored landmark studies with researchers at

Imperial College London and Johns Hopkins University that used modern brain imaging to map how psychedelics affect consciousness. She also pushed for global drug policy reform, arguing that criminalization blocked vital research and harmed public health.

Her advocacy has been both eccentric and visionary, and hers is one of the few success stories in the business of psychedelics, leading to a series of Beckley retreats and Beckley Psytech.

Back to the flameouts and pivots. Another company, First Person, a functional and psychedelic mushroom supplements maker, tried to list more than once. It ultimately withdrew its planned 2024 US IPO, a sign that public investors had cooled on consumer mushroom stories.

Optimi Health, a Canadian manufacturer focused on GMP psilocybin and MDMA, moved the other way in late 2025.[5] It filed for a US IPO to raise up to $25 million. Whether that deal works out is a real test of investor appreciation for the business of psychedelics.

The real rub is how mushrooms are perceived by investors. On one hand, nearly all of them have probably tripped in some Burning Man camp and discovered the true Return on Investment of a human soul. On the other hand, building custom drugs from what amounts to a popular commodity seems like an impossible task, especially considering the legal ramifications and cost of research. These companies are not Big Pharma, and they aren't capitalized to take advantage of scale or even popular opinion. What's more likely is that these companies sell out to Big Pharma and mushroom-related medicines begin percolating out into the wild hidden behind brand names and flashy advertising.

Ultimately, we're watching the psychedelic flameout in real time. *Willamette Week* reported in October 2025 that two listed firms that had bet on the market were heading for the exits.[6] Kaya Holdings said it would sell its interest in a large Portland "service center" and shift toward a crypto treasury play. Silo Wellness angled away from mushrooms and toward a defense focus. The reason was blunt. Their businesses were "too long term, too regulated," and not conducive for a public company that must make money for shareholders, said Kaya CEO Craig Frank. Silo, which changed its name to Born Defense and will help "end forever wars" by achieving "peace through strength." From *Willamette Week*:

> Silo's plan to build a 960-acre shroom retreat in rural Oregon near Ashland hit a wall in late 2022, CEO Mike Arnold says, when the Jackson County Planning Commission changed land-use laws to confine psilocybin facilities to commercial zones, making the rural property off-limits to psilocybin businesses.
>
> "I really had some big goals in southern Oregon," Arnold says. "But the fix was in."
>
> Now, Arnold says he wants to create an ethical defense company that invests in weapons makers that are vetted through the Just War Doctrine. First articulated by Saint Augustine, among others, the doctrine sets ethical parameters for when a nation is permitted to engage in a military conflict.

What this says about the mushroom industry is anyone's guess. It's clear, however, that there is a great deal of interest in the space from everyone, including those selfsame investors and CEOs who pivoted from mushroom retreats to, apparently, smart bombs. The question, then, is how to build a mushroom business without going to jail or ending up a caricature of the desperate CEO who switches to cryptocurrencies.

The lesson is simple. Drug development can justify public markets because the upside from a single approval can be large, even if the path is long and risky. Consumer and services start-ups struggle once the first-week headlines fade. Oregon's legal program is growing, and early data are encouraging, but the slope looks more like a slow-build public health service than a high-margin growth story, which makes it a hard fit for quarterly earnings.

If you map the winners and the wreckage, a pattern emerges. Companies with protected science, careful trials, and patient capital sometimes survive the hype cycle. Everyone else either pivots or gets priced out. In other words, the money was never in a box of mushrooms. It was in the long work of turning a compound into a medicine, or in staying private long enough to find a real business under the mulch.

Other mushroom businesses involved the process of bringing people into the world of shroomies. Retreats, sessions, and counseling appointments are now some of the most popular ways to access plant medicine, and the market is booming. Prices range from a few hundred dollars for an afternoon session to almost $9,000 for an all-inclusive resort vacation that revolves around one or two intense mushroom sessions complete with fresh vegan food, live music, and professional facilitators.

One of those people is Curtis Smith. Smith built his life around helping people see the world. For twenty years, he ran tours through Southeast Asia, Central and South America, and Europe, building a career around logistics, adventure, and connection. Then the pandemic brought everything to a halt. The pause forced him to reconsider what travel was for, and what he wanted his work to mean.

"I had a twenty-year background in the travel industry running tours all over the world," he told me from Nicaragua, where he was preparing for his next retreat. "Post-COVID, the travel business had been completely at a pause, and I had some time to sit back and reflect on how I wanted to take the next steps in life. In many ways, it was a great opportunity to make a shift."

Smith has long blond hair and a tan that shows us that he spends more time outdoors than in front of a screen. He's affable and relaxed, something that I noticed in a lot of mushroom practitioners.

Smith's shift came through plant medicine. Smith's company, Inward Travel, grew out of his own ayahuasca ceremonies, sessions that asked him to look inward and then act on what he found.

"In the same way that I had played a big part in helping people experience some of the most beautiful places on the planet," he said, "I wanted to take that to the next level with plant medicine, to go to places where they've been using these medicines for thousands of years, where the knowledge and wisdom run deep, and where people can share them in profound, authentic ways."

He said he wanted to be a bridge.

"I want to help people find those places, meet those healers, and have those experiences in safe and supported ways," he said. "And in the same ways that we'd always run tours to create great friendships and the time of your life, I wanted this to include healing too."

The pandemic pause gave him time to realign his values. He'd begun to see how much the travel industry had changed. Before, trips felt transformative; now, he said, they were often curated for Instagram. The work no longer felt connected.

"I wanted something more fresh," he told me. "Just from my own personal experience, plant medicine has been transformational and has been a guide throughout so many moments in my life."

The idea for Inward Travel arrived at a mushroom ceremony.

"It was through a ceremony that I felt that idea come up," he said. "There was this rush of excitement, and it just felt thrilling. For the first time, I was sharing something I'd always kept hidden, that I used plant medicine and that I believed in it. It felt like coming out, like saying, 'Hey, this isn't something to fear. This is something that can help everybody.'"

Plant medicine became both compass and cofounder.

"Each time I sit with psychedelics, I'm sorting through not just personal experiences and relationships but business ideas," he said. "These ideas just fly in from all directions. It's like our brains can suddenly hold a bigger framework, put the pieces together, and see from a much wider lens."

Those insights shaped Inward Travel into a company that merges traditional hospitality with sacred ceremony. Smith runs curated retreats in Peru, Mexico, and Gabon, countries where plant-medicine use is legal or unregulated. His focus is on safety and authenticity, pairing travelers with experienced shamans and facilitators. Every trip includes preparation and integration support, often guided by medical professionals.

A ten-day iboga retreat in Gabon costs about $8,000. "It's a steep fee," Smith admitted, "but the goal isn't just healing, it's to do it right." The price covers high-quality lodging, travel logistics, and collaboration with local experts like Stéphane Lasme, a former NBA player from Gabon who now helps bridge Western seekers with indigenous *ngangas*, or shamans. Other offerings, such as ketamine experiences in Mexico, are overseen by physicians on Inward Travel's advisory board.

Legal caution is built into the business model.

"My business partner is a lawyer," he said, "so it's been great to have his guidance throughout. There's certainly some risk in that, but I don't want legality to hold me back. Fear isn't really something that's come up. We offer these experiences only in countries where it's not illegal, so people can do this safely and legally."

Two years in, Smith still doesn't take a salary.

"It's been a passion project, a hundred percent," he said. "I feel fortunate that I had another career for twenty years before this that's allowed me the flexibility to spend time on something I'm passionate about. Obviously, with any business I want it to succeed and grow, but more out of its capacity to help more people."

He's clear-eyed about the ethical concerns that follow any venture built around indigenous medicine.

"We don't want to affect the integrity of the experiences," he said. "We're trying to support local shamans, preserve cultural practices, and stay small enough to keep the focus on transformation rather than expansion."

Looking ahead, Inward Travel plans to expand carefully into more interesting medicines.

"Iboga has been used there for generations, and now people in the West are learning about its power. Veterans and people with PTSD are finding healing through it. We want to help people experience it in the place where it began, with authenticity and care."

When I asked what these journeys feel like in practice, Smith smiled. "I think about the experiences that we get to have in Peru," he said. "We have shamans singing their *icaros*, which is just beyond any kind of device that can play music. You're getting this type of coding that people can perform in their *icaros* as they're sharing, really tapping into the medicine as we're experiencing it."

Inward Travel, then, isn't just about movement across borders, it's about stillness, listening, and the courage to turn the traveler's gaze inward.

Smith's vision is the simplest kind of mushroom business and the kind that still makes money. If you are planning to get rich selling psychedelic mushrooms, however, make a different plan. That is the short version. Ian Bollinger, one mushroom geneticist I spoke to, put it plainly.

"The real money's not in the mushrooms," he told me. "It's in the pickaxes."

High prices today for dried psilocybin are a by-product of prohibition, not scarcity. Once cultivation opens up, anyone with a plastic tub, a spore syringe, and YouTube can grow more than they need for a few dollars. Margins collapse and moats vanish. You cannot patent a mushroom that grows in a closet, and, even if you could, the culture will not support it.

This is what makes mushroom cultivation so interesting, and so similar to home brewing. The average home brewer could get beer cheaper at the corner store. The durable businesses sit around the edges including substrates, grow kits, testing labs, packaging, and genetics. The simple problem is that you can't create a mushroom bar the way you'd set up a beer or cigar bar. Having most of your customers nonverbal for six hours doesn't lend itself to a solid business idea.

Ian has lived this. He's in the business of analyzing mushrooms, testing grows to ensure they contain psilocybin and that they are the strain the growers claim they are. He likens it to the services that are testing THC gummies and the like, services that ensure that the contents of a pink, squishy gummy aren't poisonous or some kind of weird hybrid chemical. He helped launch the Psilocybin Cup in Oakland in 2020, persuading cultivators to submit samples for HPLC testing, then spent years in labs analyzing entheogenic mushrooms.

"I've probably tested more entheogenic mushrooms than most people on the planet," Ian said. His view on the business matches his lab data. "You could literally grow a year's worth of microdoses for about fifty bucks," he told me.

While start-ups chase brands and gummies, Ian is working on something slower and more protective. He cofounded the Entheogen Genome Foundation to sequence full genomes of psilocybin-containing fungi from around the world. The mission is defensive and simple. He wants to publish the genetic blueprints so no one else can patent the originals. You can patent a modification but you cannot patent what is already documented. He doesn't want mushrooms to fall into the wrong hands.

His genomics work complicates potency myths. Variants in the classic psilocybin gene cluster do not cleanly predict strength. "We have seen mushrooms with the exact same genes associated with psilocybin production with wildly different potencies, sometimes one to five times," he said. Environment and other pathways matter more. He prefers lineage over strain, a cleaner way to trace back to wild populations. Think Penis Envy as a lineage from Colombian Amazonian *cubensis*, with variants like Yeti or Jack Frost branching off. Some physical quirks, like mutations, are induced across many lineages and are not single-gene signatures.

This also reframes product. We eat dried mushrooms because prohibition rewarded storage and shipping, not freshness. Fresh and dried can feel different. Meanwhile, cutting-edge work has two fronts. First, there's delivery. Bollinger sees a world in which we buy transdermal patches, inhalers, and other routes that do not require eating fungi. Second, he sees value in managing cultivation inputs. He's seeing "doped substrates" that add tryptamine or even inert metals. Mushrooms are heavy-metal accumulators, so gold ends up in the fruiting body if you feed it to them. His friend, Travis Tyler Fluck, has grown shroomies on colloidal gold and gives the fruits away. Why? Because no one knows what exactly will happen when you tweak a mushroom grow with strange minerals and chemicals, and it's important for the good guys to find out before the bad guys do.

The work mixes field collecting with modern sequencing. Foragers send wild specimens, many never described in the literature. The team uses Illumina and Nanopore to assemble polished genomes. They publish a living open library. Ian calls it "genomic guardianship." It is not anti-science or antibusiness. Instead, it is a line in the sand. If a company lifts a gene from a rare African *Psilocybe* and turns it into an industrial pathway, there will be a paper trail to the ecosystem and a clear argument that benefits should flow back.

"We are not trying to punish people making money," he said. "We are trying to reward the good guys."

The tension between community and industry will follow the cannabis script. Ian remembered asking Ed Rosenthal, the so-called Guru of Ganja, what he would change about legalization.

"Nothing," Rosenthal said. Then he looked around and added a caveat. When marijuana became legal, businesses stripped away the underground feel, leaving dispensaries that looked like Apple Stores. "Where's the community now? It's almost nonexistent because it was choked out by the industry."

That is the caution. Ian's view is not antibusiness. It is anti-monopoly. "We need insulation for the community," he said. Build therapies and clinics, yes. Leave room for people to grow, gift, and guide without getting priced out or locked out. You can sell jars of sauce and still have farmers markets. His frame is guardianship rather than gatekeeping.

"These substances are powerful, like driving a car," he said. Competency and safety matter. So does preserving a path for legacy growers, facilitators, and small peer networks.

Another interesting start-up I talked to is called Safar. Safar is a good example of a "pickaxe" play. It is not growing mushrooms. It is building tools for the people who help others use them well.

"Safar translates to journey in Persian," founder Sabba Nazhand told me. He is dapper and plainspoken and wants to make money and help people. His start-up offers AI-guided coaching, including post-mushroom integration. That he is doing it with software might give some psychonauts pause, but finding a qualified integration specialist is hard, especially in a fast-growing field.

"It is an AI integration management platform, which allows practitioners, psychedelic-assisted therapists, facilitators, coaches, to create custom protocols and to manage and communicate their information with their clients," he said. The goal is simple.

"It's a two-sided AI coach. Providing insights for the practitioner and providing insights for the client," then measuring whether integration is working with "outcomes-based metrics" and validated psychological scales.

The product direction came from a gap in his own care. After a series of 5-MeO-DMT sessions in Manhattan, he walked back into life with no scaffolding.

"They gave me a hug and said have a nice day," he told me. "I was kind of disassociated for two weeks from my family, from myself, from work."

He built Safar as a last resort for folks who can't get access to a human counselor. The app captures useful signals between sessions, using voice tone, emotion, even haptics. The manifesto is clear about first principles: The tool is not the destination.

"We want to get people back to community and nature," it says. "We're not taking away from ceremony," Nazhand told me. "We're meeting people where they're at."

"Psychedelics are just tools," he said. "They open the door. It is your responsibility to go through that door and integrate."

A company like Safar allows mushroom integration to become cheaper and more accessible. While it's ideal to have a human working with you, maybe you're in a place where even integration is illegal or culturally frowned upon. When that happens, you have to depend on new tech.

When it comes to the business of shroomies, the near term looks like this: We're going to see commodity cultivation at home and folks will sell services and set standards with real margins. We're going to see software that helps people and practitioners track, pace, and integrate change. On the clinical side, AI will change the way we integrate after our trips.

Everyone I spoke to expects regulation to land with a thud and change the entire industry. Sadly, they say, pharma and the government will be involved.

"We have no choice," Nazhand said. That is another reason to build honest tools now.

As for the lab frontier, chemists will try to keep the plasticity and mute the trip, swapping groups on the molecule to change effects. Some of that will work. Some should work only inside therapy rooms. Both tracks can exist. Folks will build regulated therapy systems and leave space for the amateur with a monotub. It's definitely a new model designed for a medicine that is so strange and new that nobody yet knows how to administer it, let alone what mushroom research will bring in the next decade.

All these folks know is that something big is coming and it's not just the shroomies talking.

Purple Mystic

Just outside the sprawl of Washington, D.C., tucked in the folds of Maryland's rural fringe, a couple, let's call them Jack and Jill, hosts mushroom retreats out of their home. It's not a wellness center or a clinic, at least not yet, but a place that participants consistently describe with two words: *sanctuary* and *safety*.

Jack and Jill are tanned and tattooed. They look like typical modern tech folks who moved from the boardroom to Burning Man. They even studied computer science and business in college before they entered the corporate world. Most of their ink stopped at their shoulders so they could maintain the facade of corporate drones, but when I met them, they were ruddy and wiry from working on their farm and organizing events for their friends and neighbors.

Their journey into facilitation began not with a business plan but in a living room in Baltimore, sitting in a circle with a former anesthesiologist turned underground guide. That guide, immunocompromised from cancer treatment, once participated in a Johns Hopkins study led by Roland Griffiths, and she told them about the transformative nature of plant medicine. Jack and Jill started going to the circles out of a need to expand out of their boring, workaday worlds.

During that time, they took a few trips, and their facilitator was looking for a replacement. The facilitator herself was a mushroom convert. Her experience using and administering the medicine was so transformative that she left her medical practice to hold psychedelic space full-time, illegally, quietly, and with a reverence that appealed to her friends and clients. When COVID hit, she couldn't continue in person, so the couple stepped in, hosting retreats in their home while she facilitated over Zoom. They took on the logistics, the testing, the hosting, and the care.

What started as caretaking and taking over for a facilitator who couldn't risk exposure grew into something more. They began opening their home and land to a group of folks who wanted to get away from the Beltway and experience psilocybin in a rural setting. They started a monthly mushroom event where a few dozen folks showed up, took mushrooms, and talked. It was exactly what those people were looking for in a post-COVID world that was increasingly mediated by cellphones and conferencing apps.

Their land is beautiful. It's a farm with goats and a pair of gamboling horses. There are chickens and two big outbuildings that they are planning on converting into event spaces. When I was there, they took me down to the goat pen to meet the flock. I had always known goats were strange creatures, but to look at them with their strange horizontal pupils that afford them nearly 340-degree vision was trippy even without mushrooms.

"People love to come down here during ceremonies," they said. "They love to look at the goats."

Over time, Jill quit her corporate job at one of the FAANG companies. Jack was laid off and decided to stay that way, focusing instead on the potential of their little farm. They spend their days on the farm with the goats and their daughter.

"It became really clear that this place wants to be a place for healing," they said. "And people really respond to that."

One special place on the farm was an old oak tree they led me to. The tree, three stories tall with a full, lush canopy, had been on the property for over a century. Its roots were exposed, gnarled fingers clambering out of the earth and spreading nearly to the road.

Nestled in the roots were tiny figurines, rocks, crystals: gifts left by participants to thank the land for their spiritual experience.

"This is the center of the farm," they said. "Everyone just gravitates here."

They call their ceremonies *family-style*, and that's not marketing speak. Guests cook breakfast together, share stories around the fire, and come back months later to help clean, chop wood, or assist new guests. One participant flew in from California just to help run a weekend session. Another couple from Philadelphia, strangers when they arrived, became like kin. When I was there, a group of participants were clearing wood from the front yard, a job that was made harder by the heat and the humidity. I thought they had hired workers before a big event. They didn't. They were volunteers.

Their model is quietly radical in its simplicity: psychedelics as medicine, yes, but also community as medicine, and nature as medicine. These three pillars support the experience. Participants often show up in fuzzy socks and old hoodies, looking nothing like the wellness influencers who now dominate the psychedelic space. There is no Lululemon, just T-shirts and linen pants. They're not there for spectacle. They're there to heal.

"We're spiritual people," they said, "but we're not pushing feathers and beads. People come here and feel like they belong, even if they just left a corporate job and don't know where else to turn."

What was lovely about Jack and Jill is what makes all psilocybin facilitators fascinating: They saw a medicine that helped them and wanted to share it. They also saw their niche, part spiritual, part community, into which to slot the psychedelic experience.

Still, they are navigating the same tensions as everyone else in the space. First, they needed to maintain integrity while surviving economically. Most circles in the area charge upward of $1,100. They often start closer to $800 and even offer sliding scales. Long term, they hoped to subsidize the medicine work by opening their property midweek for corporate retreats. They are envisioning a model where companies pay to reconnect with nature and each other, while offsetting the cost for those in need of deeper healing. If the medicine ever became legal, they said, they'd consider running corporate mushroom retreats, something that might seem anathema to the buttoned-up world of business. But they both agreed that, over time, taking a bunch of mushrooms with your coworkers could be as popular as doing a ropes course.

"So, but until then, you know, I think part of what works is that we are in our home and everybody feels very much at home," said Jack. "In fact, that's one thing that, if we do build something, it's going to be really, really important to us, that it feels like a home. We think that's part of why people connect so quickly here. They really feel like family, you know?"

"The biggest thing is that people consider this a sanctuary," said Jill. "And as the weekend progresses towards the end, the word that comes up a lot is, it felt safe. We've both been in communities where it has not been safe."

Their dream includes turning the barn into a dedicated center, perhaps even under the umbrella of a church with South American roots whose founder promotes plant-medicine ceremonies. That church offers not just legitimacy but potential legal protection. Yet they're adamant that the heart of what they do can't be scaled by spreadsheets or diluted into Instagram content.

"Some of the most important medicine isn't the mushroom at all," said Jill. "It's when someone realizes they can ask for what they need and receive it. That someone else will sit with them, without needing anything in return. That changes people."

It's not for everyone. But for those ready to do the work, to sit on the floor, to eat communally, to be witnessed in vulnerability, it's often life changing. "We're not trying to help people transcend their humanity," Jill said. "We're helping them become more human."

What they offer isn't just an experience. It's a rebuttal to the commercialization that looms in the industry. "We're doing our part," Jack said, "so that if someone who's sat here ever becomes a facilitator themselves, they'll carry that reverence forward."

In a world edging toward psychedelic strip malls, these Beltway hosts are betting on something quieter: the strength of community, the power of presence, and the healing that happens when people are finally, irrevocably, seen.

Places like their farm are popping up all over the world. I would later discover that these mushroom retreats, run by amateurs and professionals alike, have become a solid way to introduce normal folks to the way of the psychonaut. And, more importantly, it's become a way to find healing and peace in a world that has become increasingly hostile.

When I went to visit Jack and Jill, I brought them a bag of my latest strain, Purple Mystic. They said they weren't ready to start growing their own mushrooms yet, so they depended on outside sources. I was happy to get rid of some of my now extensive stock.

Purple Mystic, usually shortened to PM, sits in that strange space where folklore meets the lab. The lore begins in 2008, when a forager posting on an online forum called Shroomery as Blackd0ve420 found a peculiar *cubensis* cluster in a Plant City, Florida, pasture.[1] They sent photographs and prints into the ether, and the lineage quickly picked up a mythical following for its purple-tinged cap, pancake-like shallow dome, and trips people called powerful and otherworldly.

One early Shroomery report put it simply: "The trips themselves were incredible and potent! I would experience visuals, body highs/euphoria. . . . These purple mystic (wilds) were surprisingly strong in comparison." Like most named strains of *Psilocybe cubensis*, PM is now a domesticated lineage, not a separate species, although it seemed to originally appear in the wild.

PM has tall, elegant stems with medium to large caps that can show a faint purple cast when young, then start to turn caramel in high humidity and dry to straw gold. The photos Blackd0ve420 posted showed ribs that looked outright regal with their purple spores, although, as is their wont, my homegrown shroomies didn't show off coloration. Gills run from pale to deep chocolate as spores mature. Spore prints for PM are purple-brown, standard for *cubensis* and fitting for the name.

Because the origin story points to Florida pastures after summer rain, I added a bit of humidity to my BOOMR Bin, ensuring they would get lots of moisture. The first flush fruited with tall, conical domed caps, and the second flush got wider and a little quirky.

PM, like most strains, changed over time. Cultivators cleaned up the genetics, and PM is now known for robust colonization, assertive rhizomorphic growth, and canopies that come on all at once when surface conditions are right. It tolerates beginner mistakes, recovers from slightly dry or slightly wet conditions, and shrugs off modest temperature swings. It likes to cluster, which makes for photogenic harvests and easy trims.

Reports skew bright and outward at lighter amounts, with a clean lift, warm body buzz, and a headspace that stays curious and social. Colors pop. Music bites. Outdoors feels inviting. At higher amounts, the visual field softens into geometry, and time gets rubbery.

When I tested PM, I found the trip I took to be strong at small doses, about four grams during one test. As I tested various strains, I found there were some that I could "think" under, my brain still worked, and others that forced me to lie back and simply accept the visuals and feelings. PM was one of the latter.

There are flashier names. There are lineages with stranger shapes. Purple Mystic survives because it does the simple things well. It colonizes fast. It fruits hard. It carries that warm, classic *cubensis* mood people picture for a friendly, creative afternoon on a blanket with friends. Though a modern find, it feels like rediscovering something old. A pasture surprise that moved into classic lab work without losing its character, like bringing the richness of wild orchids into a clean lab line. Today, it lives on through spore syringes carried around the world, embraced by growers who want a fast, vivid, classic *cubensis* experience.

Working with Jack and Jill and other practitioners made me think harder about why we're all turning to shroomies in our own lives. I think the answer is simple: They're a unique medicine that can do many things for many people. They're a great party tool, they're helpful when you need to solve a thorny problem, and they're helpful for folks in mental distress. I've used mushrooms to help visualize chapters of novels I've been writing and to reduce anxiety. One experience in particular stands out.

After my son left for college, I fell into a situation where I'd lie quietly in my room and just seethe with anxiety. For decades, my mental state was quiet. I never thought about much at all, simply going with whatever flow I was in. This allowed me to write eleven books (twelve, counting this one), and eleven thousand blog posts for TechCrunch. This also allowed me to sublimate nearly everything in my life under a heavy layer of eating and drinking.

When my son left, my life changed irrevocably, or at least it seemed that way. I was in a massive panic, and I felt my chest seizing up regularly, a feeling that I'd equate to a heart attack merged with heartbreak.

I went under with about four grams of Penis Envy during one session and lay there, wondering what I could do about these feelings. The mushrooms, for their part, were very agreeable.

"What's the problem?" I asked myself.

"This feeling," I answered.

Keep in mind this was all in my head. My ego was speaking to my id, my consciousness to my subconscious. Simultaneously, I was seeing wild shapes, neon tramways, wild blue and red boxes, strange faces. I saw myself as a child that needed a hug, and I tried to comfort myself.

I'd give myself the feeling. I'd think about my son, about what I had lost, about my failures. I'd let myself feel the anxiety rising.

"Is that all?" I asked myself.

"I guess?" I said.

I did it a few times, bringing up the feeling of anxiety.

And over the course of the session, I completely reduced the feeling, turned it off. It was gone in a way that seemed almost impossible only a few hours before.

That's why I think places like Jack and Jill's are so popular: They let people experience a kind of self-soothing therapy. That I was able to easily experience and learn to cope with that feeling of anxiety was amazing to me, and something I wanted to share.

Here is how I think about it. As we enter what appears to be a truly dystopian age, tools like psilocybin alongside kind, trained practitioners feel like one of the best and cheapest ways to get healthy again. That said, without proper integration, taking a bunch of mushrooms probably will not help much.

Integration is the bridge between the vision and your life. Grof put it plainly: "Successful therapy with [psychedelics] requires intimate understanding of the significance of set and setting,"[2] or those extra-pharmacological factors that shape the arc of the experience and what you carry forward from it. When the room, the people, the intention, and the care plan are aligned, the medicine stops being a random storm and becomes work you can build on tomorrow. Grof's clinical notes then move beyond the session into the morning after, recommending "a long interview," writing a detailed account, and giving space for dreams and art, all to "facilitate the integration of the material and its application to everyday life." He even cautions against reaching for sedatives at bedtime because "they also inhibit the process of natural integration of the unconscious material."

A more user-friendly, hands-on version of the same counsel shows up in Coleman's field manual. After a session, they advise you to eat lightly, rest, and, crucially, take time, because "jumping right back into your daily routine doesn't honor, or help facilitate, the deep healing process that's taking place."[3] Coleman also names a very common arc, the post-journey "contraction," where you feel less expansive than you did during the trip and might misjudge the value of the work. The advice is simple: Give it time, set a follow-up with your sitter or therapist, and let the insights percolate.

The thread running through the modern research interviews is similar. Richard Louis Miller's *Psychedelic Medicine* closes his overview with a sober reminder that there is "no such thing as a one-dose miracle cure."[4] You still need continuity, aftercare, and real behavior change for durable benefit. Even in the practical how-to discussions of set and setting, James Fadiman reduces it to controllables that support integration later, from intention to physical context. "Setting is literally the physical situation in which you find yourself," he says, quoting Hofmann's old line to choose environments that help the psyche settle and process.

Put differently, the trip is not the treatment. The treatment is what you do with the trip. In my experience collecting these sources, the consensus looks like this: Schedule time after, not obligations. Debrief in detail with a trusted guide. Write and draw before the memory gels. Watch your dreams. Move the insight into one small change you can repeat this week. If the session opens with grief or fear, do not force it closed. As Grof notes, completion and "final integration" may arrive days later, sometimes by way of a single powerful dream.

But that is the point. Integration turns an extraordinary state into ordinary, lived change. As Coleman puts it, create a "cocoon" for a couple of days afterward, get support, and give yourself permission to incorporate what you learned into your "psyche, body, and life."

So, we're close to the end of my growing journey and I've tried to answer every question I had when I started my experience. But there's one final question: Should you try mushrooms?

Modern research keeps pointing to the same conclusion. Psilocybin is a serious tool for certain mental health conditions, not a cure-all, but a catalyst. Studies now suggest that mushrooms help with depression, PTSD, anxiety, and some addictions. Recent clinical trials involving people with treatment-resistant depression have shown that a single psilocybin-assisted therapy session can significantly improve mood and well-being for several weeks.[5] The leading theory is simple enough: Psilocybin increases communication between brain networks, loosening rigid patterns of thought that keep people stuck. The real bottom line is simple: Psilocybin can reduce depression and anxiety.

Generally, mushrooms shift perception and emotion. People often describe a warm lift, deeper self-reflection, and a sense of connection to nature or to something larger than themselves. Colors and patterns can intensify. Memories surface with new context. Set, setting, dose, and personal sensitivity shape the arc, and some journeys are smooth and insightful while others can be difficult, with anxiety, nausea, or disorientation. The difference often comes down to preparation and integration afterward.

What's most interesting is the rise of community among mushroom lovers. Groups who take shrooms together tend to find community, especially if they work together after the trip. Group integration can help cement these friendships and help folks who might feel alone or have trouble communicating find solace in others.

One friend I spoke to who took mushrooms with Jack and Jill reported a sense of belonging, of well-being, and of friendship. He treats sessions at their farm as opportunities for growth and connection.

Another practitioner, Ehren Cruz, runs a community and retreat space outside of Asheville, North Carolina, called The Sparc. He was all smiles when we talked about his view of folks who took mushrooms regularly.

"It could be a very powerful and major step, but it is a step in a progressive journey. It is a step in your hero's journey. So you never want to just push in all your chips and then say, 'I need this to work in desperation.' Nor do you say, 'This is my one ticket to having a visceral spiritual experience.' You know, just embracing it as part of a continuum of your own growth is important."

"The medicine can be a very powerful opportunity to just know yourself in a more authentic and deep way and then find ways to support that with community," he said, repeating Jack and Jill's admonition that community was key. "I mean, there's a very rich, powerful, open community here too of fellow seekers and fellow people that are just ready to support the betterment of humanity."

When shouldn't you take mushrooms? And are there alternatives?

As we discussed before, there are so many factors associated with "proper" mushroom use, including set and setting and the potential mental health danger associated with psychedelic states. Mushrooms were once called psychotomimetics, the key part being "psychoto."

Taking them without preparation or supervision can be dangerous. Some start-ups are trying to change that. For example, Dillan DiNardo, CEO at Mindstate, intends to strip mushrooms of their psychedelic aspects, leaving only the tools that help with depression and anxiety.

He puts it bluntly: "We're interested in perhaps making psychedelics obsolete." His team maps how different synthetic compounds touch different receptor families, then tests combinations to see whether they can reliably evoke a single quality, like awe or empathy, without the rest of the psychedelic package. The goal is targeted, repeatable states, not a scattershot experience. He wants to formalize the medicine and take the guesswork, the set and setting, the messiness, out of mushrooms.

DiNardo, who has the swagger and dark wardrobe of a Silicon Valley founder, was a consultant who moved into health investing and finally saw the future in merging AI with medicine.

His is the "beyond the natural" thesis. Natural molecules come with complexity. DiNardo's group assays diverse synthetics against many brain targets and feeds those results into large models that link pharmacology to phenomenology. The bet is that if you can match the receptor mix to the felt effect, you can design a pill that restores, for example, a sense of beauty in someone living with anhedonia.

"When you restore that capacity to see the beauty in the everyday," he told me, "It's a mountaintop experience. You don't need the drug every day. The perspective tends to stick."

"We study the mechanisms at many different molecular, cellular, psychological, neural levels. Ultimately, we don't understand the mechanism, but what seems to happen is that there is this perspective shift. So someone who, for example, has had depression for decades, all of a sudden looks around at their daily life and they remember again that they love life, right?"

DiNardo also wants to make pharmaceuticals that mimic the effects of mushrooms, in that you can take them once and never do another trip again.

"They don't necessarily need to take that drug again every day for the rest of their lives. Having been to the top of the mountain and seen what it's like at the top of the mountain, that perspective shift kind of stays with you. So that's what we see sometimes with some psychedelics, and that's what we want to really bottle in pill form and make much more reliably accessible."

Regulators will have the final say. The company is in phase one now, with early human data expected in 2026, and years to go before any approval. The focus is medical, not recreational, though it is hard to ignore what this kind of control could mean for psychotherapy and, eventually, wellness. If their vision lands, mental health care changes shape. Fewer blunt instruments. More precise tools that help people access empathy, awe, or motivation on demand, then carry those changes into ordinary life.

None of this replaces the basics. Whether we are talking about classic psilocybin journeys or new targeted compounds, outcomes still hinge on intention, support, and the work people do afterward. There is no one-dose miracle. There is a set of tools, some ancient and some still being built, that, used with care, can help people move again.

That's what folks like Jack and Jill and Ehren Cruz are building out on their farm, goats included.

Fatback

The plane banked hard and landed soft. As we waited on the tarmac, a thin mist of water vapor drifted through the air-conditioning vents while I looked out over a landscape of royal palms and blue mahoe. Heat pressed against the window. Beyond the runway, the hills were a deep, heavy green, the kind of color that tells you everything grows fast here. I was in Montego Bay, Jamaica, for a multiday retreat. The four-day event included two psilocybin ceremonies under the strict guidance of facilitators and health professionals from Beckley Retreats, the group connected to Lady Amanda Feilding.

The timing felt almost suspiciously perfect. Back home, I had been living inside this book for months, closing out chapters, moving paragraphs around, trying to cram years of work into clean, linear sections. I had grown more mushrooms than I could ever count. I had gone on multiple trips, some tender, some rough. I had talked to almost a hundred people, scientists and shamans, growers and chemists, start-up founders and cautious therapists, pulling apart every angle of mushrooms I could find, from Mesoamerican rites to designer capsules sold in glossy packaging to make us happier or crack open something we might call a religious experience.

What I did not have, at least not recently, was time with the medicine without a recorder running. Every conversation had turned into material. Every personal insight got filed under "possible chapter opening." I was starting to feel less like a person and more like a reporter trapped inside a draft. So, when I stepped off the plane and felt the thick Jamaican air hit my face, it felt like a small reset. For five days I would not be the guy asking questions or chasing citations. I would be another person in a circle, taking tea from a cup, breathing, waiting for the caps and stems to come up and do their quiet work. I needed a break with the shroomies before I could finish writing about them.

The noise of the airport would have been lovely if I had not been in such a mood. Reggae blasted from tinny speakers over the baggage carousel, and a few attendants were dancing as they dragged suitcases off the belt. People were laughing, greeting each other, already in vacation mode. I stood there with my carry-on, feeling like I was made of sandpaper.

The months before the retreat had been rough. My day job as a cryptocurrency marketer, a role I had never liked in the first place, was slowly slipping away, and my homelife felt frayed at every edge. I was tired, short tempered, and not much fun to be around. I stopped microdosing because I was worried about what it was doing to my brain. A lot of what the shroomies had taught me—stop drinking, be a better father, let yourself be happy—had started to fade under the weight of old habits and new stress. It was like the lessons were written on a whiteboard and someone had slowly wiped them away with the back of a hand. It turned out that microdosing had been helping and that stopping was silly.

At the JetBlue terminal, I ordered a Bloody Mary and knocked it back too fast, trying to summon the old version of myself, the one who was big and angry and drunk and pretending that counted as being alive. It did not work. The drink sat in my belly like a stone and all I got for my trouble was a flare of acid reflux and a quiet sense that I was out of tricks.

Now, on the ground, I was just angry.

Being a journalist had been a blast. Whenever I traveled, someone picked me up at the airport and dragged me to a faceless hotel where I'd check in, dump my bags, and then watch movies, masturbate, and work. I figured this trip would be more of the same.

I harrumphed my way out of the terminal and tried to find my ride, texting the team at Beckley like a spoiled toddler that I couldn't see him anywhere.

The team, to their credit, responded firmly.

"He's there. Look for him," they wrote.

They were not there to coddle me.

I found him standing by a white van near the curb. I kept my heavy leather jacket on, even in the thick Jamaican heat, as if I needed the armor. He stepped forward at once and offered to take my bag. He was a big, jovial man with a sly smile and careful eyes, the kind of driver who has seen too many tourists show up confused and full of themselves.

We drove in silence for a while, the air conditioner fighting a losing battle against the humidity. My shirt began to stick to my back. Out the window I could see bright houses, tin roofs, and kids in school uniforms walking along the road. At some point he glanced over and asked where I was from.

"New York," I said.

"I lived there once," he replied. "I'll never go back."

I believed him. The island was lush and loud and bright. Trees the color of oregano crowded the hillsides. Houses were painted in joyful shades of turquoise and yellow. Smoke curled from small cookshops by the road. Life was clearly hard here, but people moved with a kind of easy rhythm. Most faces held a smile, or at least were ready to offer one if you met their eyes.

I, on the other hand, had no smiles to give. I stared out the window and let my mind chew on old anger. We drove for about thirty minutes before turning onto a narrow dirt road hemmed in by trees. The van rattled and shook. A few KFC buckets and plastic bottles hid in the underbrush, the usual human stain. The cynic in me snorted. All this beauty, and they still throw trash on it.

Farther up and farther in, the road climbed in slow turns. We spent another thirty minutes on that track before coming to a gate set in the middle of a wide pasture. A horse paddock ran along one side of the drive, a few animals flicking their tails in the heat. The road wound through a stand of trees and up toward low hills. The gate read GOOD HOPE in iron letters.

It was so on the nose it made me wince. Hope was exactly what I had come looking for, and exactly what I did not trust. I shifted in my seat, hot in my jacket, feeling the old part of me roll its eyes while another quieter part, the one that had booked this trip in the first place, leaned forward as the gate swung open.

At the top of the hill we reached a rambling white house with a roof of black tile. The van stopped with a soft hiss of brakes, and the air felt thick and green after the ride. A woman in the Good Hope uniform walked up to the door and opened it before I could reach for the handle.

"Welcome to Good Hope," she said. "We'll take your bags to your room and I'll show you around."

Good Hope began in the mid eighteenth century as a sugar estate along a bend in the Martha Brae River, first granted to Colonel Thomas Williams. Later John Tharp took it over and turned it into a two-thousand-acre plantation. He became one of the largest landowners and slaveholders in Jamaica, working the property with thousands of enslaved people. The guide did not rush this part. She described the cane, the mills, the river, the people forced to live and die here. The house looked quiet, but the history under it was not.

After emancipation, the estate shifted into a small village that housed and employed former plantation workers. The Georgian great house and outbuildings watched over cane fields and cattle pens. Over time the roofs gave way, walls cracked, and the place slid toward ruin.

Now the land is a retreat, an eco-style resort with a wide kitchen, a countinghouse turned into a small bedroom, and a carriage house cut and rebuilt into guest rooms. It only holds a few dozen people at a time. The great house sits above the grounds. Ceiling fans turn. The grass is trimmed. I listened, or tried to, as the guide walked me from room to room, naming the original furniture and mirrors, noting which boards were old and which were new. She told me how the great house once had holes in the roof where vines pushed through into the bedrooms. Now the wood was polished, the plaster fresh. The wild growth had been pushed back outside.

She handed me a glass of coconut water.

"This is from our trees," she said. The drink was cold and faintly sweet. She added that an Ugli fruit would be waiting in my room, also picked on the grounds. I nodded, thanked her, and kept walking through the bright restored rooms.

It is hard to say much about my time at the retreat, because you are told not to. The first thing the facilitators explained was that they were building a "container," a held space for the group. Once that space is set, they said, everything that happens inside it belongs to the people in it. Stories stay in the room.

There were ten other people with me. Each one carried something heavy. Grief. Fear about the future. Old trauma that would not let go. Illness. A mind that would not slow down. We sat together at meals and before sessions, trading hints of our lives without giving too much away. I knew just enough to feel their weight and to respect it.

Because of that, I will keep to broad strokes. I will write about what happened to me, what I saw in my own head and felt in my own chest, and leave their stories alone. The details that belong to others are not mine to hand over.

What I can say is simple: Everyone who came to Good Hope walked in with one set of problems and walked out with another way of seeing them. No one left untouched. The place, the work, the people, shifted something in each of us, even if I can't tell their full stories out loud.

Meanwhile, I was just angry. Angry at my crumbling career, at a family that felt like it was slipping into some new shape without asking me, at the holidays rolling toward me again with their yearly reminder that my father was gone. The whole thing sat in my chest like a stone.

I went straight to my room, dropped my bag, and lay down on the bed. The ceiling fan turned slowly. Outside I could hear distant voices and the scrape of a rake on gravel. Inside there was nothing. No email. No kids shouting from the next room. No sirens. Just a thick quiet that felt almost fake at first, like a soundstage version of peace. I stared at the ceiling and let myself stop moving.

The retreat had a loose frame around that quiet. There were a few required group sessions and three meals a day. Breakfast, lunch, and dinner, all at long tables where we were meant to sit together and pretend we were not already judging each other. In the early mornings they offered movement classes, some blend of stretching and dance. I avoided them without much guilt. I preferred coffee and sitting on the veranda, letting my mind chew on its own problems instead of my hamstrings.

In the afternoons we had breathwork. That I did. We lay on mats, eyes closed, while a facilitator talked us through patterns of breathing that felt awkward at first, then strange, then oddly powerful. My hands tingled. My chest felt tight, then loose. I began to see what they were trying to do. They wanted to get us out of our usual grooves, to pull us a few inches away from panic and habit so we would be ready for the trips ahead.

The staff were all professional coaches, not robe-wearing gurus. One of the coaches even grew mushrooms for a living and talked about strains the way some people talk about wine. A small Jamaican woman with a quick smile turned out to be a singer. She slipped into song in between giving instructions. There was a jazz drummer on-site, hired to play during our sessions, ready to push and pull the mood as we went under.

Around them moved a larger crew. Cleaners who swept the verandas before sunrise. Cooks who slipped quiet plates of food in front of us. Porters who carried bags and refilled water jugs without fuss. People who seemed genuinely glad we were there. Their work held the whole place together so the rest of us could fall apart in relative comfort.

The first trip came on the second day. We started the morning with smoothies, light and sweet, and were told not to eat again until after the trip, around two in the afternoon. That small rule made the whole day feel sharper. Every hour stretched. I knew what was coming, or thought I did. Most of the group did not.

I fell into the worst possible role. I was the guy who had read too much and done too little. I heard myself explaining the difference between cubes and cyans, talking about potency, talking about grams and body weight, talking about "come up" and "peak" and "integration." I went on about how the dose was carefully measured, how the staff had done this many times, how we would probably feel at different points in the day. I spoke like I knew the script. Inside, I knew I was bluffing. I had no real idea what this would feel like in my own body.

That is the strange comfort of these retreats. They give you an extremely controlled space to meet the medicine. You are not in a basement with a random bag from a friend. You are in a place with staff who check on you, nurses who know your name, and facilitators who ask about your fears before they hand you anything. Everyone arrives with a different story, but everyone wants the same thing. To feel safe. To be held in a container that will not fall apart when things get hard.

So the place becomes a mix of resort and clinic. You eat good, simple food. There is no booze and no late-night bar scene. People sit by the pool and talk quietly instead of shouting over music. You go to sleep early. In the morning you stretch on yoga mats under slow fans while someone burns incense in the corner. The staff lays out blankets, eye masks, and small plastic buckets, practical little signs that this is not just vacation.

You get soft towels, filtered water, and a schedule printed on nice paper. You get a polite reminder to write down your intention before the session starts. You get a nod from the facilitator, who promises to stay with you if things tilt sideways. You also get a carefully weighed bowl of mushrooms. In the end that is the deal. A pleasant resort, a medical shell around it, and inside that shell, a handful of fungi that are about to rearrange the day.

My first trip there was four grams of a local strain called Fatback. It was a Jamaican cube strain based on another strain called Fat Ass. Fatback started as an offshoot of the Fat Ass strain and has been shaped over years of growing. It is not subtle. People report strong, detailed visuals with both eyes open and closed, patterns and scenes that feel layered rather than chaotic. It has become the strain most people ask for in Jamaica because it tends to sit in a sweet spot, intense but not wild, a trip that feels full without knocking you off the planet.

I went into this trip loaded with expectations. The dose was about what I was used to, so I treated it like familiar ground. I picked a spot near the drum kit so I could feel the music in my chest and not just in my ears. Before we took anything, they handed out little slips of paper and told us to write our intentions. I wrote something like "Less fear" and "Less stress." I knew even then that they were vague wishes, not real honesty. My brain had other plans.

On the way to Jamaica, I had already started breaking the rules. In the airport terminal I bought a drink to calm myself, and with that I also picked up a duty-free bottle of rum. At the retreat they were very clear. No alcohol. No edibles. No sleeping pills. The point was simple, they did not want anything else in your system when the mushrooms hit.

I nodded along when they explained it, then ignored them. That first night I poured a few glasses of rum and told myself it would help me sleep. Instead, I lay in bed listening to the frogs. They were everywhere, a whole chorus starting at dusk and never letting up. In Brooklyn I could sleep through trash trucks at three in the morning and cars blasting techno under my window. That chaos read as home. Out in the dark with the frogs, I felt exposed, like the whole island was awake.

The more I tried to force sleep, the further it drifted. I shifted on the lovely mattress, counted breaths, listened to the ceiling fan ticking as it turned. The rum dulled the edge but did not quiet my head. Under the frogs and the fan, I could feel a low anxious buzz building, the sense that I had already stepped wrong before the real work even started.

By the time morning came and we lined up for smoothies, I was tired, wired, and pretending to be calm. I told myself the dose was familiar and the setting was safe, that I could manage whatever came. But between the lack of sleep, the cheap rum, and the polite little card that said "Less fear" in my own handwriting, I had already given the trip plenty to work with.

We took the medicine in tea. They measured out our doses, stirred them into warm cups, and told us that "booster" doses would be offered later if we needed them. It had the feel of a small ritual. Not church, but close. The facilitators spoke softly, touched shoulders, checked in with each of us before we drank. They kept everything light and kind and almost tender. I sat there with my usual private weather system of gloom and dread and tried to match their smiles.

The session was supposed to last six hours. I told myself I had been here before, that the dose was familiar, that I knew the territory. I lay down near the drums again, pulled the blanket up to my chest, and waited.

I was not ready.

When the first waves hit, they did not ask permission. Fractal patterns began to roll in behind my eyes, growing more complicated the harder I tried to make sense of them. I did what I always try to do when things get rough. I started talking to myself, the way you talk to a frightened kid. I told the scared, twitchy part of my brain that everything was fine, that it was only chemicals and time, that I had been through this before and it would pass.

To keep my mind from spinning out, I used my old alphabet trick. Think of an animal for each letter. A was aardvark, B was bear, C was cat. I walked through the list like I had many times before, a quiet chant for my own benefit.

The drummer was working all of our nerves. He was not playing songs. He was building a soundscape that sat on top of our thoughts and pressed down. He had an ocean drum full of beads that he would tilt and roll, slowly, so it sounded like wind mixed with metal. Not quite the sea, not quite static, just this restless hiss in the corner of the room.

Every minute or so he would strike three tones in what felt like a random order. They were in tune and, in any normal setting, they would have sounded like the chime of an elevator closing or a polite little alert. In this context they set my brain on fire. The notes were too clean, too sharp, cutting right through whatever pattern I was trying to build in my head.

The sounds went on for hours. Three notes. The beads washing around the drum. The fan buzzing in the dusk. My thoughts sliding around, never quite landing. It felt almost impossible to grab on to anything solid while my brain rattled in my skull and those three tones kept dropping in like small, bright hammers.

At the time I hated it. Later, when I could think again, I understood why it worked, especially for early trips.

Three tones are simple enough for a mind on mushrooms to follow, even when that mind is frightened. There is no real melody to get lost in, no big emotional swell that drags you into some long story. It is just a short pattern. Your brain starts to expect it. You know it is coming back. That small bit of predictability is a kind of rope.

For people who are new to this, that matters. In the first hour of a trip, anxiety is at its peak. Your sense of time is bending. Your body feels strange. A full song, with lyrics and big shifts, can pull you in ten directions at once. Three tones do something else. They give you a clear, repeatable anchor. You can breathe with them. You can count them. You can tell yourself, "When the chime comes again, I am still here."

The sound of the beads fills the space between the tones without grabbing the center of your attention. It is like a low wash that keeps the room from feeling empty. The fan adds another constant line. Together they hold the room in a narrow band: not silent, not overwhelming, just dense enough that your thoughts have something to push against.

So while those chimes annoyed me in the moment, they did their job. They carved a steady shape into the chaos, something basic and clear that even a scrambled mind could track. For early trips, when people are trying not to bolt from the mat or sink into panic, that kind of simple, repeating pattern can make the difference between feeling trapped in noise and feeling held by sound.

The trip kept pressing in.

I saw my family. Not as clean snapshots, more like scenes slipping in and out of focus. I saw my wife, the way her eyes sometimes slide past me, tired, distant, or simply done. I saw my mother and my grandmother, judging me. I saw my kids, and with them all the ways I had fallen short, all the sharp words, all the times I had chosen work or escape instead of being present. Each memory arrived like a small indictment. I felt the pressure of tears rise and stop in my throat. Instead of crying I squeezed harder on the alphabet, like it was a string of beads I could pray on.

At some point, a blue face appeared, built out of thin lines of light, hovering in the dark behind my eyes. My breathing went shallow. Lying on my back felt like too much, like gravity was helping the mushrooms run straight into my spine. I rolled onto my side and curled up, knees tucked in, a tight little knot on the mattress, trying to lessen the impact of the sensory flood.

Then a voice came through the noise. Calm, casual, almost amused.

"You're going to be fine, buddy."

It was the voice of a close friend, someone I love and respect, someone who, in real life, has seen me at my worst and did not run. For some reason she was right there in my head, steady, talking to me like we were sharing a coffee instead of a psychedelic crisis. She kept saying versions of the same thing, that I was safe, that this would pass, that I did not have to fight every single image that came up.

Underneath the visuals and the self-reproach, something else started to rise. It was not comfortable, not at first. More like a widening view. I could see my family again, but this time not only as people

I had failed, but as people who had stayed. My kids, still running into the room, still asking for me. My mother and grandmother, who had carried me further than they ever admitted. Even my own tired, flawed self, still trying.

By the end of that first session, shaken and wrung out, I could see what the trip had really been pushing toward from the start. It was never about "less fear" or "less stress." Those were small words I wrote to make myself feel like I had a handle on things. The core of it was simpler and harder. It was about seeing how much I already had, and how rarely I let myself feel grateful for any of it.

The blue face. My friend's voice in my head. The steady reminders that I was safe. All of it pointed to the same blunt message. "You should be more grateful." Grateful for your wife. Grateful for your kids. Grateful for your family. Grateful for what your father gave you all those years ago, before he wasted away in a bed talking about ethereal deer. I needed to be grateful for the fact that I was even still here, breathing on a mat in a room full of strangers who were also trying to fix something inside themselves.

Even this book snapped into focus. I could see what it needed from me. Not just facts and quotes and a neat history of spores and species. It needed my own mess in it. My doubt and shame and surprise. I kept thinking, nobody really knows what they are doing with mushrooms yet, not in any deep way, except perhaps the cultures and healers who have been passing down their stories from generation to generation and who shared with me their knowledge willingly and with love. If I was going to write about them, I'd have to show what they did to me, not hide behind science and stories. The gratitude was not only for the people in my life, but for the fungus itself, for this odd, stubborn gift that had wandered into my midlife crash and decided to rearrange the furniture.

Then my body went cold. Not a gentle chill but a slow, creeping cold that started at my feet and hands and moved inward. I pulled the thin retreat blankets up to my chin and tried to burrow into the mat. The colors began to fade a little. The sharp edges of the visuals softened, like someone turning down the contrast. I lay back and let the mushrooms drain out of my nervous system inch by inch.

The end of that trip came early for me. It was like the tide turning before I was fully ready to leave the water. I felt wrung out, but also relieved. Fatback, whatever mix of history and chemistry it carried, was strong. Stronger than I had planned for. I had walked in acting like a veteran and walked out humbled. I was glad to come down.

Around me, the rest of the group was crawling back into themselves in their own strange ways. One person sat up and complained that he had not felt anything at all. They looked annoyed, like a customer sent the wrong drink. Another person lay on their back grinning, eyes wide, explaining that dead relatives had come to sit with them, like it was the most normal thing in the world. Someone else had spent the middle of the session in full project manager mode, talking nonstop to the facilitators, asking them to move chairs a few inches, to adjust pillows, to change the music, to clear space for "better flow."

During the peak of my own trip, that chatter had driven me mad. Every request snapped me out of my fragile focus. I wanted to tell them to shut up and lie down. As the night went on, and the heavy part of the medicine eased off, the whole scene shifted. The bossy voice, the endless requests, the small parade of staff shifting furniture while a room full of half-melted adults lay around in eye masks, it all turned ridiculous in the best way.

The music came up and one of the facilitators began to sing, the strange three-tone music that the jazz drummer was playing falling away into something beautiful. He was on guitar, others were on drums and shakers. Everyone was swaying to the music.

It was from an old folk song:

Hold him Joe, hold him Joe
Hold him Joe but don't let him go
Hold him Joe, hold him Joe
Hold him Joe but don't let him go

The donkey want water (hold him Joe)
Spring 'round the corner (hold him Joe)
The donkey want water (hold him Joe)
Everybody want water (hold him Joe)

As her voice rose I started on a new alphabet. I used people's names instead of animals. A for Asia. B for Bob, my father. C for Charlie, my old jazz guitar teacher. M for Milla. K for Kasper. G for Guthrie. R for Richie. P for Pamela. A string of people, all connected to my heart. I went through that alphabet repeatedly, this time sending little bursts of love to each of those folks. I knew they wouldn't feel them, but I knew that I felt them, and that's all that mattered.

By the time the session wound down, and people started trading stories in low voices, I could feel a thin layer of warmth under the exhaustion. We were all ridiculous. Terrified, hopeful, broken in private ways, and still willing to hand our minds over to a handful of dried mushrooms to see what might shake loose. For me, that first day, what shook loose was one clear thing. Be grateful.

The next day we were all a little brittle. The team took some of us to a small private beach. I joked that I might try to find a margarita or two. It felt like the right old habit to reach for. Unfortunately, we were too far from any bar and the only thing on offer was warm tap water. My urge to lean on self-destruction was thwarted again, this time by simple geography.

The night before I had sweated through my pajamas. For whatever reason my body answered the mushrooms with a light fever, heat without any real flu symptoms. It was strange and I did not want to repeat it, so I turned the air-conditioning up and tried to let my body settle.

I had taken to visiting the frogs that kept me up all night. I found the tiny tree frogs that had been tormenting me. They were Jamaican laughing frogs, each no more than an inch long. What they lacked in size they made up for in volume. They wailed through the darkness with a sound as sharp as a car alarm, their small bellies pulled tight with air. Nearby I found a family of bullfrogs that spent their days basking in the sun and their nights burping out a slow, patient song. I should have hated the noise, but something shifted. I began to depend on these amphibious neighbors. Their presence grounded me, and I was looking forward to visiting with them after my second trip.

We spent part of the day doing simple breathing exercises. We were told to breathe rhythmically and fully for nearly forty-five minutes. I was sure it would be silly and dull. Instead I found myself hissing through my mouth, pushing air out through my nose in time with yoga music, watching my chest rise and fall. At some point I realized that I had not paid real attention to my breathing in years. My breath moved on its own while I worried about everything else. Sitting there on that mat, lungs working like bellows, I could feel how tight I usually kept myself and how strange it felt to just sit, breathe, and do nothing else.

The day passed and I felt better. I was more social, lighter on my feet, and a little more willing to joke with people. Even the staff noticed that I was smiling. "When you first came here, you were so sad," said the woman who had given me the tour a few days before. Hearing that stung a bit, because she was right, but it also felt like proof that something had shifted. In this intense setting, the shroomies were doing what they were supposed to do, they were loosening the knot I carried around my chest.

The next morning it was time for my second and final session. A facilitator sat with me beforehand and asked how much I wanted to take. They told me that, if I felt able, I should try to push the envelope a little and lean into the work. This time we were taking Monster Mac, a popular Jamaican strain built from the equally popular Melmak Penis Envy line. People there talked about it with a kind of respect, a mushroom that grows in thick, oversized fruits with a neat brown cap that looks almost harmless. It is also loaded with psilocybin, which I would soon learn in my own body. I agreed to the higher dose and tried to steady myself for whatever came next.

The process was the same as before. I picked a spot farther from the speakers and drank the tea. About thirty minutes later I felt a wave of pressure in my stomach and knew I had to stand up and go to the bathroom. One of the facilitators took my hand and walked me through the lush grounds, past the little frog pool, to the tiny concrete outhouse at the edge of the property. Inside, the light was dim and flat. I looked down at the floor and watched it come alive. The concrete began to swirl in tight, shifting patterns that I had never seen before. It stopped looking like concrete and started to look like clear water over a shallow pond lined with small stones. For a moment I expected to see fish moving in the current. I sat quietly on the toilet, staring at the floor and wondering what, if anything, I should do next.

A few minutes later I walked back toward my mat. The entire landscape looked different. The trees seemed to vibrate in place, their outlines trembling. The fan in the corner no longer hummed, it screamed. The sound buzzed in my ears like a sheet of metal being struck over and over. The music felt worse than the night before. It sounded off-key and sharp in a way that made my teeth hurt. Every sound pressed in at once. I lay back on my mat, closed my eyes, and felt a terrible thought drop into place. I was not at a retreat. I was in rehab.

I became convinced that the entire retreat existed to get me clean from alcohol. In that moment it all seemed obvious. Someone had reached out to me with this offer. I had accepted, but in my mind it had all been orchestrated by my boss at the crypto job I was about to lose. Everyone, from my family to the facilitators, was in on it. We were all there to get clean from something. The couple in the circle became suburban wine drunks. Other people, in my head, turned into heroin or pill addicts. I was just a standard boozer who had finally been cornered.

I lay there stunned. There were no visuals now, just an overwhelming absence of normal thought. I could only imagine and reimagine the supposed process. They pick you up at the airport and tell you not to drink. They put you in a place with no mixers, no sugary drinks to sneak whiskey into. They give you good food, then mushrooms, then make you sit through a grueling session to scrape you clean.

I was burning up with heat. Earlier that day I had picked up a small shell from the frog pond. I held it in my fingers, turning it over and over, staring at it and breathing deeply the way they had taught us. It was the only thing I could manage. The shell became my anchor, something solid in a mind that felt like it was coming apart.

They had given me six grams, which was probably why I had dropped into this level of psychedelic experience. I felt stunned, stupefied, and paranoid all at once. This was ego death, or close enough. I could not think. I felt my mind pull away from my body while this imagined rehab machine did its work on me.

In the middle of the trip, I reached up toward the mushroom farmer and grabbed his hand. I whispered to him, ashamed. I asked him to take the bottle of rum out of my room.

"I understand this all now," I said.

"Of course you do," he said, kindly.

This was delirium tremens in my mind. This was withdrawal. I told myself I was feeling what people feel when someone takes their heroin or their pills away. I believed I was being stripped down to nothing. I felt trapped in a kind of private hell, and the only thing I could do was endure it and keep going.

Time moved in weird ways. I held the little shell in my hand and stared at it as if it were the only solid thing left in the world. I stayed with my breath. I stayed with the shell. Slowly the rhythm around me began to shift. The music softened and lost its sharp edges. The atonality eased and something gentler rose in its place. Colors settled. Sounds stopped tearing at me. The world began to come back into view. The fire in my mind, which had roared, started to cool. I could feel myself returning, inch by inch, as the heat drained out of me and the panic loosened its grip.

A song came out of nowhere, sung by angels or devils or spirits or the frogs themselves.

"Don't worry 'bout a thing," someone sang. The guitar followed and so did the drums. The night opened.

I heard myself singing along, as loudly as I could, as the night enveloped this strange little band of adventurers in that dark Trelawny jungle.

Home

I wish I could say the mushrooms broke me of my boozing. I wish I could say they fixed my relationships, made me a happier person, and turned me into a better father. They did not. Even my rehab fantasy—that someone loved me enough to spend thousands on my health, that someone saw my pain and wanted to heal me—was a fantasy, generated whole cloth out of the trip. I called friends and family after that last trip and they were completely flabbergasted.

I had made it all up.

But maybe it was for the best. My brain had concocted a madcap effort to get me to stop drinking too many Negronis at open mic night at my local pizza place. It worried about me or, rather, I worried about me. I knew that I couldn't keep drinking like I had been drinking, even in my curtailed, post–fat journalist state. It reminded me that it probably wasn't healthy for me to buy cheap duty-free rum and sneak it into a health resort. So it gave me something I couldn't get from anyone else in my life: fear, perspective, and—again, I shudder at the self-help language—self-awareness. Mushrooms are just mycelium that rise out of manure or torn up soil, part of a quiet system whose whole job is to share resources with a connected network that has been working for millions of years.

It's what our brains do with the mushrooms that makes them important.

When we eat shroomies we get a brief chance to tap into that long, strange past and to make a different choice about our future. After all my events, all my research, and all my attempts to use mushrooms as a cure for my sadness, I learned something hard and simple. All they could really do for me was clear some space in my head, the way a decluttering specialist clears out a hoarder's rooms. The trip wipes the shelves clean and leaves you standing in an empty house. What you bring back in afterward is up to you.

After that, I stopped drinking at home and chose to drink only in social settings. I tried to smile more and listen more. When a friend told me about a traumatic experience from his past, I felt tears rise and I pulled him into a hug, which is not my usual move. I made a point of playing with my kids instead of lecturing them. I went to more live music performances. I tried to do things that gave me real pleasure rather than chasing the same old habits that only reinforced my pain. The mushrooms did not save me. They gave me a clear space to land. The work of living differently was still mine.

Each trip also gave me the opportunity to enjoy some brain plasticity. Right after a strong mushroom trip there is a strange quiet in the system. The storm is done, but the clouds are still moving. Brain cells are not rewired from scratch, but they do enter a more flexible state. Animal-focused research with classic psychedelics shows more dendritic spines, more synapse growth, and changes in the receptors that sit on those synapses. Human work, with brain scans and blood markers, hints at the same trend. Circuits that were locked into rigid loops of rumination and fear are a little less stuck. You could call it a temporary "wet cement" phase. Old grooves are still there, but they are easier to step out of.

The period after a mushroom trip feels strange because the mind is still open. Researchers now suggest that psilocybin triggers a short burst of neuroplasticity, a time when the brain can shift old patterns and begin to lay down new ones. In plain terms, the mind becomes easier to teach. It is a window when habits loosen, fears quiet down, and new ways of thinking can take root with less resistance. This does not last long. It tapers over a week or two. Still, it is enough time for a person to choose a different path if they are willing to work at it. The drug does not carry you. It only clears the clutter so you can see where to step.

A study in *Nature*[1] explains things a little more clearly:

> Neuroplasticity can be investigated at multiple levels of analysis. At the molecular level, it comprises changes in gene and protein expression, as well as post-translational modifications. Of particular importance is brain-derived neurotrophic factor (BDNF), a neurotrophin that regulates neuronal growth and synaptic plasticity. Changes in gene and protein expression give rise to morphological changes, including the formation and modification of synapses and dendrites. In particular regions, most notably the hippocampus, neuroplasticity also comprises neurogenesis. These processes modify neural circuits, ultimately manifesting in learning, memory, and changes in adaptive behavior. Neuroplasticity is crucially activity-dependent at the cellular level, which translates into experience-dependence at the level of cognition and behavior: people learn both passively and actively from their experiences, adjusting patterns of thought, emotion, and behavior accordingly.

In other words, there is a small but definite change in the brain after a trip, and clinicians try to use that window to change behavior. For a week or two after a session many people reported that habits felt less automatic. New behaviors feel more possible. Simple things, like going for a walk, cooking a meal, or calling a friend, land with more weight. Therapy can go deeper because the story about "who I am" is less rigid. The point is not that the drug heals you on its own. The point is that it opens a stretch of time when effort has a higher return.

That window closes in about four weeks. Plasticity does not stay high forever, and life rushes back in. What you do in those days matters. If you use them to rest, to talk, to write, to set small honest goals, the new patterns have a better chance of holding. If you run straight back into the same grind, the old loops are waiting. Mushrooms can tilt the brain toward change for a while. The work of building a different life in that softer clay is still yours.

And it was still mine.

People call mushrooms medicine. They call trips "doing the work." The old me would have scoffed at that. How is lying around on a yoga mat work? How is listening to EDM medicinal? How can these little dried things keep me from walking in front of a Chicago city bus?

But, little by little, they showed me that they were all those things. They were helpful, medicinal, and vital. They altered my brain and they altered the brains of countless others I interviewed for these chapters. They opened my eyes to a new way of thinking about the brain, about personality, about anxiety, and about depression.

And they helped me feel better.

This book began in the dark and ended in the light. As I type these words I am looking out over Ohio Street in Chicago, about a mile from where I first wanted to take my life. The sun is shining, the rain is gone, and the world is a little better. Not perfect, just better. All because of a little baggie of poop-loving shroomies and a choice to keep going, to do the work, and to take the medicine.

It was enough to make this jaded, cranky journalist want to smile again. My hope, ultimately, is that it could someday do the same for you.

Acknowledgments

First, I'd like to thank Greg Ferenstein for starting me down this road. He saw an exhausted, cynical, burned-out man and tried to help. For his wisdom and care I'm forever grateful.

I'd also like to thank P, the moderator who ran my first event and many of the events that followed.

I'm deeply grateful to the wonderful staff at Good Hope in Jamaica, as well as the excellent counselors, musicians, and growers associated with Beckley Retreats. It is customary to maintain anonymity when it comes to facilitators. Otherwise, I would gladly share their names and contact information because they were that good.

Thanks to those who helped me protect my mental health, including Dr. Nittenberg and PB.

I'd also like to thank my early readers, including the people who reached out when I published the first chapter in my newsletter. Your kind words reduced the sting of sharing something so personal.

Thank you to my agent, Alice Martell, who helped shepherd so much of my work. Special thanks to Daniela Rapp at Skyhorse, who took my idea and helped me run with it. I've never worked with an easier editor.

Thank you to my family, including Nina. I do all this for you.

Thank you to my father, for showing me how to live with joy and die with dignity.

And thank you to the shroomies.

References

Chicago

1 Centers for Disease Control and Prevention (CDC), "Suicide Data and Statistics," National Center for Injury Prevention and Control, last modified 2023, https://www.cdc.gov/suicide/statistics/index.html.

Meet the Shroomies

1 Hawksworth, David L., and Robert Lücking, "Fungal Diversity Revisited: 2.2 to 3.8 Million Species," *Microbiology Spectrum* 5, no. 4 (2017), https://doi.org/10.1128/microbiolspec.FUNK-0052-2016.

2 Popkin, Gabriel, "'Wood Wide Web'—the Underground Network of Microbes That Connects Trees—Mapped for First Time," *Science*, May 15, 2019, https://www.science.org/content/article/wood-wide-web-underground-network-microbes-connects-trees-mapped-first-time.

3 Allegro, John M., *The Sacred Mushroom and the Cross* (New York: Doubleday, 1970).

4 Jacobsen, Rowan, *The Truffle Hound: On the Trail of the World's Most Seductive Scent, with Dreamers, Schemers, and Some Extraordinary Dogs* (New York: Bloomsbury Publishing, 2021).

5 Beiler, K. J., D. M. Durall, S. W. Simard, S. A. Maxwell, and A. M. Kretzer, "Architecture of the wood-wide web: Rhizopogon spp. genets link multiple Douglas-fir cohorts," *New Phytologist* 185, no. 2 (2010): 543–53, https://doi.org/10.1111/j.1469-8137.2009.03069.x.

6 Jacobsen, *The Truffle Hound*, 147.

7 Stamets, Paul, *Mycelium Running: How Mushrooms Can Help Save the World* (Berkeley, California: Clarkson Potter/Ten Speed, 2011), 11.

8 Loron, Corentin C., Corentin François, Rachel H. Rainbird, and others, "Early Fungi from the Proterozoic Era in Arctic Canada," *Nature* 570 (2019): 232–35, https://doi.org/10.1038/s41586-019-1217-0.

9 Hobbie, Erik A. and C. Kevin Boyce, "Carbon Sources for the Palaeozoic Giant Fungus Prototaxites Inferred from Modern Analogues," Proceedings of the

Royal Society B: Biological Sciences 277, no. 1691 (2010): 2149–56, https://doi.org/10.1098/rspb.2010.0201.

10 Lanfranco, Luisa, Paola Bonfante, and Andrea Genre, "The Mutualistic Interaction between Plants and Arbuscular Mycorrhizal Fungi," *Microbiology Spectrum* 4, no. 6 (2016), https://doi.org/10.1128/microbiolspec.FUNK-0012-2016.

11 Baker, R. P., and Arturo Casadevall, "Fungal Proliferation Before and After the Cretaceous–Paleogene Mass Extinction in North America," *bioRxiv preprint*, published December 12, 2025, https://doi.org/10.64898/2025.12.11.693767.

12 Sheldrake, Merlin, *Entangled Life: How Fungi Make Our Worlds, Change Our Minds & Shape Our Futures* (New York: Random House, 2021), 156.

13 Hinneburg, Hannes, Shanna Gu, and Gita Naseri, "Fungal Innovations—Advancing Sustainable Materials, Genetics, and Applications for Industry," *Journal of Fungi* 11, no. 10 (2025): 721, https://doi.org/10.3390/jof11100721.

14 Sheldrake, *Entangled Life*, 167.

15 Averesch, Nils J. H., Graham K. Shunk, and Christoph Kern, "Cultivation of the Dematiaceous Fungus Cladosporium sphaerospermum Aboard the International Space Station and Effects of Ionizing Radiation," *Frontiers in Microbiology* 13 (2022), https://doi.org/10.3389/fmicb.2022.877625.

16 de Bekker, Charissa, William C. Beckerson, and Carolyn Elya, "Mechanisms behind the Madness: How Do Zombie-Making Fungal Entomopathogens Affect Host Behavior to Increase Transmission?" *mBio* 12, no. 5 (2021): e01872-21, https://doi.org/10.1128/mBio.01872-21.

The Wise Woman and the Banker

1 Reynolds, Hannah T., Vinod Vijayakumar, Emile Gluck-Thaler, Hailee Brynn Korotkin, Patrick Brandon Matheny, and Jason C. Slot, "Horizontal Gene Cluster Transfer Increased Hallucinogenic Mushroom Diversity," *Evolution Letters* 2, no. 2 (April 1, 2018). https://doi.org/10.1002/evl3.42.

2 Stamets, Paul, *Psilocybin Mushrooms of the World: An Identification Guide* (Berkeley: Ten Speed Press, 1996), 16.

3 Stamets, *Psilocybin Mushrooms of the World*, 4.

4 Gartz, Jochen, *Magic Mushrooms Around the World: A Scientific Journey Across Cultures and Time: The Case for Challenging Research and Value Systems* (Los Angeles: LIS Publications, 1996), 80.

5 Ibid.

6 Letcher, Andy, *Shroom: A Cultural History of the Magic Mushroom* (New York: Ecco, 2007), 26.

7 Ibid., 74.

8 Sahagún, Bernardino de, *Historia general de las cosas de Nueva España: el Códice Florentino*, 1577, World Digital Library, Library of Congress, https://www.loc.gov/item/2021667837/.

9 Durán, Diego, *The History of the Indies of New Spain*, trans. Doris Heyden (Norman: University of Oklahoma Press, 1994), 427.

10 Wasson, Valentina Pavlovna, and R. Gordon Wasson, *Mushrooms, Russia, and History, 2 vols*. (New York: Pantheon Books, 1957), 44.

11 Letcher, *Shroom*, 90.

12 Wasson, R. Gordon, "Seeking the Magic Mushroom," *Life*, May 13, 1957, 100–120.

13 Author's rendition based on P. Bahn, N. Franklin, & M. Strecker (Eds.), *Rock Art Studies: News of the world* (Vol. 3). Oxford, UK: Oxbow Books. "Amanita muscaria in

the household, beliefs, rituals, and art of the peoples of the North." Sibirskie istoricheskie issledovaniya. 46–58. 10.17223/2312461X/11/5.
14 Batyãnova, Elena Petrovna and Mikhail Mokovich Bronshtein. "Mukhomor v bytu, verovaniyakh, obryadakh, iskusstve narodov Severa." *Sibirskie istoricheskie issledovaniya* 2016, no. 1 (2016), 46–57. https://cyberleninka.ru/article/n/muhomor-v-bytu-verovaniyah-obryadah-iskusstve-narodov-severa/viewer.
15 Wasson, R. Gordon, *Soma: Divine Mushroom of Immortality* (New York: Harcourt Brace Jovanovich, 1968), 24.
16 Feeney, Kevin M., *Fly Agaric: A Compendium of History, Pharmacology, Mythology & Exploration* (Ellenburg, Washington: Fly Agaric Press, 2020), 77.
17 Bogoras, Waldemar. *The Chukchee. Publications of the Jesup North Pacific Expedition*, vol. 7. (Leiden: E. J. Brill, 1904–1909).
18 Fatur, Karsten, "The Henbane Hypothesis," *Tea Assembly*, issue 7, accessed February 9, 2026, https://www.tea-assembly.com/issues/7/the-henbane-hypothesis.
19 Letcher, *Shroom*, 32.
20 Taylor, Rogan, "Who Is Santa Claus? Santa Takes a Trip," *Sunday Times Magazine* (London), December 21, 1980, 8–10, 12, 17.
21 Morgan, Adrian, "Who put the toad in toadstool?" *New Scientist*, December 25, 1986. 44–47.
22 Hutton, Ronald, *Shamans: Siberian Spirituality and the Western Imagination* (London: Hambledon and London, 2001), 13.
23 Ibid.
24 Letcher, *Shroom*, 82.
25 Wasson, "Seeking the Magic Mushroom."
26 Tonet, Aureliano, "That Time the CIA Tested Hallucinogenic Mushrooms," *Le Monde*, August 31, 2022, updated September 5, 2022, https://www.lemonde.fr/en/summer-reads/article/2022/08/31/that-time-the-cia-tested-hallucinogenic-mushrooms_5995365_183.html.
27 Amezcua, Lourdes, "Maria Sabina and the Holy Children," *Shroom Tales*, January 24, 2021. https://www.lourdesamezcua.com/shroom-tales/maria-sabina-andtheholychildren.
28 Letcher, *Shroom*, 90.
29 Wasson, R. Gordon, Albert Hofmann, and Carl A. P. Ruck, *The Road to Eleusis: Unveiling the Secret of the Mysteries* (Berkeley, California: North Atlantic Books, 2008), 31.
30 Wasson, *The Road to Eleusis*, 33.
31 Hofmann, Albert, *LSD, My Problem Child: Reflections on Sacred Drugs, Mysticism, and Science* (Sarasota, Florida: Multidisciplinary Association for Psychedelic Studies, 2005), 17.
32 Bogenschutz, Michael P., "Psilocybin-Assisted Treatment for Alcohol Use Disorder: A Randomized Clinical Trial," *JAMA Psychiatry* 79, no. 10 (2022): 953–62, https://doi.org/10.1001/jamapsychiatry.2022.2096.
33 NYU Langone Health, "Psychedelic Drug Therapy May Help Treat Alcohol Addiction," December 28, 2022, https://nyulangone.org/news/psychedelic-drug-therapy-may-help-treat-alcohol-addiction.

How Do They Work?

1 Redhead, Scott, Moncalvo, J. M., Vilgalys, R., Matheny, P. B., Dávalos, Laura, Guzmán, Gastón (2007). "Proposal to conserve the name Psilocybe (Basidiomycota) with a conserved type," *Taxon*, 56. 255-257. 10.2307/25065762.

2 Schäfer, Tim, Fabian Haun, Bernhard Rupp, and Dirk Hoffmeister, "Dissimilar Reactions and Enzymes for Psilocybin Biosynthesis in Inocybe and Psilocybe Mushrooms," *Angewandte Chemie International Edition* 64, no. 46 (2025): e202512017, doi:10.1002/anie.202512017.
3 Earle, Franklin Summer (1906), "Algunos hongos cubanos." *Información Anual Estación Central Agronomica Cuba* (in Spanish), 1: 225–42 [240–41].
4 Singer, Rolf, *The Agaricales (Mushrooms) in Modern Taxonomy*, Waltham, MA: Chronica Botanica, 1951.
5 Gartz, *Magic Mushrooms Around the World*, 29.
6 Maffly, Brian, "Psychoactive Psilocybins Evolution in Magic Mushrooms," *@theU*, University of Utah, February 27, 2018, https://attheu.utah.edu/facultystaff/psychoactive-psilocybins-evolution-in-magic-mushrooms/.
7 Johnson, Bryan (@bryan_johnson), X (formerly Twitter), February 7, 2025, https://x.com/bryan_johnson/status/1988064701075648776.

Golden Teacher

1 Kings County District Attorney's Office, "More than 250 Pounds of Illegal Psychedelic Mushrooms with a Street Value of Almost $2 Million Seized from Major Grow House in Sheepshead Bay," December 16, 2016, https://www.brooklynda.org/2016/12/16/more-than-250-pounds-of-illegal-psychedelic-mushrooms-with-a-street-value-of-almost-2-million-seized-from-major-grow-house-in-sheepshead-bay/.
2 Letcher, *Shroom*, 18.
3 Pollan, Michael, "Opium, Made Easy," *Harper's*, April 1997.
4 Oss, O. T. and O. N. Oeric, *Psilocybin: Magic Mushroom Grower's Guide. A Handbook for Psilocybin Enthusiasts* (Berkeley, CA: Quick American Archives, 1976), 7.
5 Nicholas, L. G., and Kerry Ogamé, *Psilocybin Mushroom Handbook: Easy Indoor & Outdoor Cultivation* (Oakland: Quick American, 2006.), 35.
6 Cornell University, "Biohybrid Robots Controlled by Electrical Impulses from Mushrooms," August 2024, https://news.cornell.edu/stories/2024/08/biohybrid-robots-controlled-electrical-impulses-mushrooms.
7 *Joe Rogan Experience*, "#1035—Paul Stamets," PodScribe, accessed February 12, 2026, https://podscripts.co/podcasts/the-joe-rogan-experience/1035-paul-stamets.
8 "Fanaticus Chronicles." Mycotopia Forums: Board Rules and Historic Threads. Accessed February 12, 2026. https://forums.mycotopia.net/board-rules-historic-threads/95-fanaticus-chronicles.html.
9 Letcher, *Shroom*, 279.

Stargazer

1 Davis, Alan K., et al., "Effects of Psilocybin-Assisted Therapy on Major Depressive Disorder: A Randomized Clinical Trial," *JAMA Psychiatry* 78, no. 5 (2021): 481–89.
2 Ross, Stephen, et al., "Rapid and Sustained Symptom Reduction Following Psilocybin Treatment for Anxiety and Depression in Patients with Life-Threatening Cancer: A Randomized Controlled Trial," *Journal of Psychopharmacology* 30, no. 12 (2016): 1165–80.
3 Carhart-Harris, Robin L., et al., "Trial of Psilocybin versus Escitalopram for Depression," *New England Journal of Medicine* 384 (2021): 1402–11.

4 Allegro, John M., *The Sacred Mushroom and the Cross: A Study of the Nature and Origins of Christianity Within the Fertility Cults of the Ancient Near East* (London: Hodder & Stoughton, 1970).
5 Lam, Lydia, "23-Year-Old Singaporean Dies After Falling from Fifth Floor Bali Hotel Room," *The Straits Times*, May 8, 2017. https://www.straitstimes.com/asia/se-asia/23-year-old-singaporean-dies-after-falling-from-fifth-floor-bali-hotel-room.
6 Moore, Tina, Jamie Schram, Priscilla DeGregory, and Chris Perez, "Man Jumps to His Death after Taking Magic Mushrooms," *New York Post*, May 23, 2016. https://nypost.com/2016/05/23/man-jumps-to-his-death-after-taking-magic-mushrooms/.
7 Adam R. Winstock et al., *Global Drug Survey 2017: Global Overview and Highlights* (London: Global Drug Survey, 2017).

Penis Envy
1 Morris, Hamilton, "A Nice Thick Uncut 12 Inch Shroom," *Hamilton's Pharmacopeia Blog*, accessed February 19, 2026, https://hamiltonmorris.com/blogs/news/a-nice-thick-uncut-12-inch-shroom.
2 Basidium Equilibrium, "Penis Envy," Patreon, October 18, 2024, https://www.patreon.com/posts/penis-envy-114217140.
3 Prochazkova, Luisa, Josephine Marschall, Dominique Patrick Lippelt, Neil R. Schon, Martin Kuchař, and Bernhard Hommel, "Cognitive and Subjective Effects of Psilocybin Microdosing, Results from Two Double-Blind Placebo-Controlled Longitudinal Trials," *Neuropharmacology* 283 (February 1, 2026): 110722, https://doi.org/10.1016/j.neuropharm.2025.110722.
4 Harman, Willis W., Robert H. McKim, Robert E. Mogar, James Fadiman, and Myron J. Stolaroff, "Psychedelic Agents in Creative Problem-Solving: A Pilot Study," *Psychological Reports* 19, no. 1 (1966): 211–27.
5 Fadiman, James, *The Psychedelic Explorer's Guide: Safe, Therapeutic, and Sacred Journeys* (Rochester, Vermont: Park Street Press, 2011).
6 Ibid., 185.
7 Waldman, Ayelet, *A Really Good Day: How Microdosing Made a Mega Difference in My Mood, My Marriage, and My Life* (New York: Knopf, 2017).
8 Prochazkova, Luisa et al., "Exploring the Effect of Microdosing Psychedelics on Creativity in an Open-Label Natural Setting," *Psychopharmacology* 235, no. 12 (December 2018): 3401–13, https://doi.org/10.1007/s00213-018-5049-7.

Jedi Mind Fuck
1 L'Heureux, T. J., "Arizona Study of 'Jedi Mind Fuck' Magic Mushrooms Clears FDA Hurdle," *Phoenix New Times*, March 28, 2025. https://www.phoenixnewtimes.com/news/arizona-study-jedi-mind-fuck-mushrooms-clears-fda-hurdle-21468350/.
2 Ibid.
3 Baylor College of Medicine, "STARLIGHT (State-Funded Trial Assessing Recovery and Long-term Impact of Guided Psilocybin for Healing Trauma)," Baylor College of Medicine Healthcare Clinical Trials, accessed February 24, 2026. https://www.bcm.edu/healthcare/clinical-trials/h-50300.
4 Simpson, Stephen, "With Rick Perry's Backing and $50 Million from the State, Texas Set to Become a Leader in Psychedelics Research," *Texas Tribune*, June 11, 2025. https://www.texastribune.org/2025/06/11/texas-psychedelics-ibogaine-treatment-addiction-rick-perry-funding/.

5 Grof, Stanislav, *Realms of the Human Unconscious: Observations from LSD Research* (New York: Viking Press, 1975).

Blue Meanie

1 Laussmann, Tim, and Sigrid Meier-Giebing, "Forensic Analysis of Hallucinogenic Mushrooms and Khat (Catha edulis Forsk) Using Cation-Exchange Liquid Chromatography," *Forensic Science International* 195, no. 1–3 (2010): 160–64, https://doi.org/10.1016/j.forsciint.2009.12.013.
2 Coleman, R., *Psychedelic Psychotherapy: A User Friendly Guide to Psychedelic Drug Assisted Psychotherapy*, 2nd ed. (London: Transform Press, 2017).
3 Letcher, *Shroom*, 315.
4 Barba, Tommaso, Hannes Kettner, Caterina Radu, Joseph M. Peill, Leor Roseman, David J. Nutt, David Erritzoe, Robin Carhart-Harris, and Bruna Giribaldi, "Psychedelics and Sexual Functioning: A Mixed-Methods Study," *Scientific Reports* 14 (2024): Article 2181, https://doi.org/10.1038/s41598-023-49817-4.
5 Grof, Stanislav, *LSD Psychotherapy: The Healing Potential of Psychedelic Medicine, 4th ed.* (Ben Lomond, California: Multidisciplinary Association for Psychedelic Studies, 2008), 240.
6 Ibid., 251.
7 Coleman, *Psychedelic Psychotherapy*, 102.

Illusion Weaver

1 Griffiths, Roland R., Robert Jesse, William A. Richards, Matthew W. Johnson, Nathan D. Sepeda, Anthony P. Bossis, and Stephen Ross, "Effects of Psilocybin on Religious and Spiritual Attitudes and Behaviors in Clergy from Various Major World Religions," *Psychedelic Medicine* 3, no. 4 (2025): 172–91, https://doi.org/10.1089/psymed.2023.0044.
2 Griffiths, Roland R., Matthew W. Johnson, Michael A. Carducci, Annie Umbricht, William A. Richards, Brian D. Richards, Mary P. Cosimano, and Margaret A. Klinedinst, "Psilocybin Produces Substantial and Sustained Decreases in Depression and Anxiety in Patients with Life-Threatening Cancer: A Randomized Double-Blind Trial," *Journal of Psychopharmacology* 30, no. 12 (2016): 1181–97, https://doi.org/10.1177/0269881116675513.
3 Pollan, Michael, "This Is Your Priest on Drugs," *The New Yorker*, May 26, 2025, https://www.newyorker.com/magazine/2025/05/26/this-is-your-priest-on-drugs.
4 Grof, Stanislav, *The Way of the Psychonaut: Encyclopedia for Inner Journeys* (Albuquerque, New Mexico: MAPS, 1994).
5 Stevens, Jay, *Storming Heaven: LSD and the American Dream* (New York: Grove Press, 1987).
6 Griffiths, Roland, interview by *The New York Times Magazine*, "Roland Griffiths on Psychedelics and His Own Mortality," *The New York Times*, April 3, 2023, https://www.nytimes.com/interactive/2023/04/03/magazine/roland-griffiths-interview.html.
7 Aaronson, Scott T., et al., "Single-Dose Psilocybin for Depression with Severe Treatment-Resistant Depression: An Open-Label Trial," *Journal of Clinical Psychopharmacology* (2025), https://pubmed.ncbi.nlm.nih.gov/39741440/.

Wavy Caps

1 Wakefield, E. M., 1946. "New or Interesting British Fungi," *Transactions of the British Mycological Society* 29: 141–66.

2 Beaty Biodiversity Museum, "Psilocybe cyanescens—Wavy caps," Mushrooms Up! Edible and Poisonous Species of Coastal BC and the Pacific Northwest, accessed March 2026, https://explore.beatymuseum.ubc.ca/mushroomsup/P_cyanescens.html.

3 Schumaker, Erin, "Psychedelic Medicine CEO Eyes Chances under MAHA," Politico, *Future Pulse* newsletter, August 6, 2025. https://www.politico.com/newsletters/future-pulse/2025/08/06/psychedelic-medicine-ceo-eyes-chances-under-maha-00494736.

4 "Amanda Feilding, Eccentric Countess Who Backed Psychedelic Meds, Dies at 82," *The New York Times*, June 15, 2025. https://www.nytimes.com/2025/06/12/science/amanda-feilding-trepanation-dead.html.

5 "Optimi Health Files to Raise up to $25 Million in SEC Filing," *FirstWord Pharma*, September 7, 2025, https://firstwordpharma.com/story/5995377.

6 Effinger, Anthony, "Two Companies Betting on an Oregon Shroom Boom Pivot to Other Businesses," *Willamette Week*, October 1, 2025, https://www.wweek.com/news/2025/10/01/two-companies-betting-on-an-oregon-shroom-boom-pivot-to-other-businesses/?utm_source=chatgpt.com.

Purple Mystic

1 Shroomery, "Blackd0ve420's Gallery," Shroomery Message Board. Accessed March 5, 2026. https://www.shroomery.org/forums/usergallery.php/gallery/189685/screen/2.

2 Grof, *LSD Psychotherapy*, 110.

3 Coleman, *Psychedelic Psychotherapy*,14.

4 Miller, Richard Louis, *Psychedelic Medicine* (Rochester, Vermont: Park Street Press), 12.

5 Raison, Charles L., et al., "Single-Dose Psilocybin Treatment for Major Depressive Disorder: A Randomized Clinical Trial," JAMA 330, no. 9 (2023): 843–53. https://doi.org/10.1001/jama.2023.14530.

Home

1 Calder, Amy E., and Gregor Hasler, "Towards an Understanding of Psychedelic-Induced Neuroplasticity," *Neuropsychopharmacology* 48, no. 1 (2023): 104–12. https://doi.org/10.1038/s41386-022-01389-z.

Index

Please note that page numbers in italics indicate illustrations.